Also by Gail (Davis) Galvan

Diary of an American Covid-19 Era Survivor
Problematic President—Dangerous Dictators
Texting: Smash-ups, Mishaps, and Laughs
Skelly the Skunk Saves Freedom Day
On the Literary Road with a Valpo Writer
Affinity for Rainbows: Sunshine Finish Lines
New Jack Rabbit City: Starring the Chicago Hares
(with a co-author)
A Nonviable Option: Suicide? Not!
Self-Publishing Sucks Sometimes and Here's Why
(But Don't Give Up!)
Autoimmunity Counterattack: A Sequel/
The Healthy Road Back (2005, non-profit)
Autoimmunity Counterattack (2003, non-profit)
Author Unknown, Author Undaunted
Affinity for Rainbows (2002 Edition)
Autobiography of an Allergic/Asthmatic Survivor
(2001, revised edition 2014)
Paycheck to Paycheck:
Pre and Post Millennium Style
In Parents We Trust
Sneezing Seasons (1999)

Books with other poets/writers:

Write-On, Hoosiers: Celebrating Thirty Years
Banta's Banter: Savory Senior Recipes
Horizon Spectrum
Poetry Palace: Boys and Girls Clubs (2010)*
Poetry Palace (2005)
HS-Hoosier Storybook (2004)
HS-Hoosier Storybook (2002)
*(Note: No affiliation with Boys and Girls Clubs of America)

SNEEZING SEASONS
2013

The Inside Story about
Allergies and Immunology

(Told by a friendly antibody)

Written

by

Gail Galvan

SNEEZING SEASONS

The Inside Story about
Allergies and Immunology

by

Gail Galvan

Original version edited by: Sharon Radetsky-Hampal

Original graphics of Henry and George were created and

illustrated by: Michael Rasmussen

Revised graphics of the cover design and Henry and

George by: Michael Evanouski

Text by: Gail (Davis) Galvan

Originally published in 1999 by Infinitypublishing.com
862 West Lancaster Avenue
Bryn Mawr, PA 19010-3222

ISBN-13: 978-1484106310

Printed in the USA

DEDICATION

Dedicated to the creative and healthful spirit that lives within us all, my dear mom, dad, brothers and sister, with love, and—of course, dear medical researchers, and doctors, especially mine, who care.

ACKNOWLEDGMENTS

First, thanks be to God for everything, especially all of my healthy comebacks.

I wish to express my sincere appreciation to many people who offered guidance, encouragement, and assistance in preparation of this story: To Sharon Radetsky-Hampal for her editorial help and genuine insight regarding the allergy/asthma problem, the late Dr. William E. Rhodes, for his warm heart, creative energy and philosophical wisdom, Anne Hatcher, R.D., Ed.D., for her support and nutritional expertise, and the late Mr. Roy Raney from, the currently named, National Jewish Health in Denver, Colorado for his important insight after reviewing an early draft.

Thanks also to Mr. Michael Rasmussen for first bringing the hero antibody characters, Henry and George, artistically, to life and M.E. for his graphic revision. I'm grateful to Joan M. Kolodziej and Vivian Vican at Nerdworld, for their word processing/formatting skills and extra effort for the 1st edition. Fabulous job! Of course I take credit for any errors, since the book has been revised.

A final draft is the accumulation of an idea which connected with a variety of serendipitous and purposeful chain of events throughout its entire development. Thank you all for helping build the fragmented parts of *Sneezing Seasons* and making the book whole.

Special credit and thanks also to author Dr. Ronald J. Glasser, for his book, *The Body Is The Hero*, 1976, 1979, and the Amazon Kindle edition, 2012. Now you know where I got the idea to *show* the immunological war that happens within and *tell* the inside story.

Seems to me I also recall memories of watching miniature humans in a submarine traveling around inside a human body in distress. So I'd better thank those responsible for the *Fantastic Voyage* movie and story, too. This would include: Harry Kleiner, David Duncan, Isaac Asimov, Otto Klement and Jay Lewis Bixby.

Grateful acknowledgment goes out to Infinity Publishing in Pennsylvania for the initial paperback version of *Sneezing Seasons*. One of my literary dreams, this book, came to life because of you—a pioneering, innovative company offering print on demand services to unknown, as well as already established, writers.

For the latest version(s), I have self-publishing gurus and authors to thank for their continued inspiration, and publishers like Amazon and Smashwords which enable writers to make their dreams come true. What a special gift you have provided to so many unknown, yet undaunted writers. Again, our books live because of you! Also, to Ebooklaunch.com and John, for being there, thanks!

To Bruce, my amazing computer tutor, thanks for trying to teach me rather than simply solving baffling problems.

To my master website, graphics designer and storyteller friend, Michael Evanouski, from: www.golivestudios.net for all the help, encouragement, and inspiration for the last year—it made all the difference. I must also thank Wickersham, Mike and Lori's cat, for the adorable pose! Five Star Publications loved you too! Thanks so much to Five Star for the Honorable Mention for Best Cover Design (Purple Dragonfly Book Awards, 2013).

Alas, heartfelt thanks to Dr. Kansal, Dr. Katherine M. Poehlmann, for the forewords, and clker.com for all interior images. Eternal thanks to all of my colorful contributors!

CONTENTS

Dedication
Acknowledgments
Table of Contents
Foreword
Preface and Introduction

CHAPTER

1.   Marin
2.   Barb and Tim
3.   Kevin
4.   Captain Rodz
5.   The Allergy/Asthma Scope
6.   Sara
7.   The Clinic
8.   Henry and George
9.   The Work-Up Room
10.   George's Imagination
11.   Major Borline
12.   Clara and Bret
13.   The Hike
14.   The Enemy
15.   Kicking Back
16.   Henry's Feelings
17.   The Emergency
18.   Final Thoughts

EPILOGUE: A Whole New Chapter in My Life

ABOUT THE DOCTORS:

Dr. Katherine M. Poehlman
Dr. J. K. Kansal and Dr. Max Samter

SOURCES

FOREWORD by Doctor Jatinder K. Kansal

When the book, *Sneezing Seasons*, was presented to me by one of my patients, who happened to be a friend of the author, I first noticed the cover. I saw the cat on the cover and thought about all the problems so many hypersensitive people, adults and kids, have with cats and other animals, substances, and foods—patients I see every day. They have to put up with daily triggers that really should *not* be causing reactions; but they do. I noticed the word immunology in the title, also, instead of simply asthma, and again, I thought the book was right on target due to the fact that immunological disease covers the broader topic and problem relating to unlucky hypersensitive individuals. So when Ms. Galvan asked me if I would consider reading it and writing a foreword, I agreed.

From the first chapter on, I realized that this was a different kind of book and perspective. Henry, an antibody, tackles the topic of anaphylactic shock, one of the cases he is "assigned" to. A girl he likes dies from a bee sting, so as the story unfolds, it's clear that Henry is on a mission to educate other antibodies. Convince them NOT to overreact because that's exactly what happens within allergic individuals.

An immunological disease results from a disorder of the immune system. There are various categories: allergic diseases, immune complex diseases, autoimmune diseases, and immunodeficiency disorders. The most common types of allergic diseases occur when the immune system responds to a false alarm. In an allergic person, normally harmless substances such as: house dust, pollen, or foods are mistaken for threats and get attacked. This is pointed out in case after case in the book.

The principal antibody who participates in allergic reactions is called immunoglobulin E, or IgE. As Henry, an IgE antibody, goes from assignment to assignment, within human bodies, he goes about explaining how inner "wars" break out because the antigens arrive on the scene, and then the antibodies are programmed to attack. Once set into motion, unless the antibodies back off, as Henry pleads them to do, the allergic reaction flares and subsequently causes the mast cells to release the aggravating chemical—histamine. The allergic reaction then runs its course, and/or the victim counterattacks medically.

In autoimmune diseases, the medical situation gets even more serious and complicated. (Autoimmunity is addressed in the epilogue.) The body begins to manufacture T cells and antibodies directed against its own cells and organs. Misguided T cells and *autoantibodies*, as they are known, cause many very serious diseases.

I think the author, by way of Henry, does a very good job of helping people understand what's going on inside an allergic human body. When a bee stings, antibodies overreact. In one case, a crisis results from an overreaction to walnuts. (Food allergies continue to be a very significant, even life-threatening, problem for many children and adults.) This story helps people understand just how serious it can be.

The statistics for people who suffer with allergies, asthma, and/or autoimmune diseases near the end of the book, are very alarming, but, again, right on target. One message the author and I, as well as anyone in this field will attest to, is that with increased awareness, better health education and disease management (including immunotherapy/desensitization), unnecessary tragedies can be prevented. I think that's what "Henry," is trying to do. Stressing the point that if hypersensitivity is brought under control, quality of life can be greatly improved. Not only that, but essentially, lives can and must be saved.

Best Regards,
Dr. J. K. Kansal (9-13-13)

PREFACE

"For those who sneeze, wheeze, itch, swell up and feel miserable at times, I want you to know you are not alone. There are many millions who share similar agony and frustration. Though your common affliction may invade your life, alter your temperament, and turn your body into a battlefield, immunological equilibrium is still within your grasp.

Just believe that each day, every moment that you fight against sickness and work conscientiously toward wellness, makes a difference. Setbacks will come, but the bad days and moments will disappear as the clouds part ways. LOOK FOR THE RAINBOW AFTER THE RAINFALL. Follow the sun and you will be okay. Good luck from Henry and the rest of us. Also, anything medically incorrect in my book—go ahead and blame Henry."

Gail Galvan, L.P.N.
B. A. Health and Wellness Education
Metropolitan State University, Denver, Colorado

INTRODUCTION

To hopefully help increase awareness and a better understanding of allergies and immunology, for those not as familiar as others, I have included a list of terms related to the story. It might help to have handy access to the following site while reading the book: http://en.wikipedia.org/wiki/Main_Page. With the insertion of a word and one simple click, you can look at definitions. I have, however, included some of the most important terms here.

I am also going to introduce you to some of the main characters, so you will know who and what they are when their names come up, especially during the human-body-inner-immunological-wars that Henry is trying to win in order to save lives.

GLOSSARY

allergy is a hypersensitivity disorder of the immune system.[1] Allergic reactions occur when a person's immune system reacts to normally harmless substances in the environment.

allergen is a type of antigen that produces an abnormally vigorous immune response in which the immune system fights off a perceived threat that would otherwise be harmless to the body.

antibody (Ab), also known as an **immunoglobulin** (Ig), is a large Y-shaped protein produced by B cells that is used by the immune system to identify and neutralize foreign objects such as bacteria and viruses. The antibody recognizes a unique part of the foreign target, called an antigen.[1][2]

antigen is the substance that binds specifically to the respective antibody.

autoantibody is an antibody (a type of protein) manufactured by the immune system that is directed against one or more of the individual's own proteins. Many autoimmune diseases are caused by autoantibodies.

autoimmune diseases arise from an inappropriate immune response of the body against substances and tissues normally present in the body.

autoimmunity is the failure of an organism in recognizing its own constituent parts as *self*, thus leading to an immune response against its own cells and tissues.

anaphylaxis is a serious allergic reaction that is rapid in onset and may cause death.[1] It typically causes a number of symptoms including an itchy rash, throat swelling, and low blood pressure. Common causes include: insect bites/stings, foods, and medications.

asthma (from the Greek ἄσθμα, *ásthma*, "panting") is a common chronic inflammatory disease of the airways characterized by variable and recurring symptoms, reversible airflow obstruction, and bronchospasm.[2] Common symptoms include wheezing, coughing, chest tightness, and shortness of breath.[3]

B cells belong to a group of white blood cells known as lymphocytes, making them a vital part of the immune system. B cells can be distinguished from other lymphocytes, such as T cells and natural killer cells (NK cells), by the presence of a protein on the B cells outer surface known as a B cell receptor (**BCR**). This specialized receptor protein allows a B cell to bind to a **specific**

B cells (con't) antigen. The principal functions of B cells are to make antibodies against antigens, to perform the role of antigen-presenting cells (APCs), and to develop into memory B cells after activation by antigen interaction. The abbreviation "B", in B cell, comes from the bursa of Fabricius in birds, where they mature. (Latin: *Bursa cloacalis* or *Bursa fabricii*) The bursa is present in the cloaca of birds and is named after Hieronymus Fabricius who described it in 1621.[1]

cell is the basic structural, functional and biological unit of all known living organisms. Cells are the smallest unit of life that is classified as a living thing, and are often called the "building blocks of life".

corticosteroids are a class of chemicals that includes steroid hormones naturally produced in the adrenal cortex of vertebrates and analogues of these hormones that are synthesized in laboratories. Corticosteroids are involved in a wide range of physiological processes, including stress response, immune response, and regulation of inflammation, carbohydrate metabolism, protein catabolism, blood electrolyte levels, and behavior. Prednisone is an example of a synthetic corticosteroid drug that is particularly effective as an immunosuppressant drug. It is used to treat certain inflammatory diseases (such as moderate allergic reactions) and (at higher doses) some types of cancer, but has significant adverse effects. Because it suppresses the immune system, it leaves patients more susceptible to infections.

cytokines (secreted proteins and signaling molecules) the term "cytokine" has been used to refer to the immunomodulating agents, such as interleukins and interferons. They are regulators of host responses to infection, immune responses, inflammation, and trauma.[2

desensitization (also known as allergen immunotherapy) is a method to reduce or eliminate an organism's negative reaction to a substance or stimulus. Cellular level administration of small doses of toxin produces an IgG response which eventually overrides the hypersensitive IgE response.

eosinophil granulocytes, are white blood cells and one of the immune system components responsible for combating multicellular parasites and certain infections in vertebrates. Along with mast cells, they also control mechanisms associated with allergy and asthma.

epinephrine (also known as **adrenaline** or **adrenalin**) is a hormone and a neurotransmitter.[1] Epinephrine has many functions in the body, regulating heart rate, blood vessel and air passage diameters, and metabolic shifts; epinephrine release is a crucial component of the fight-or-flight response of the sympathetic nervous system.[Due to its vasoconstrictive effects, adrenaline is the drug of choice for treating anaphylaxis. Allergy[6] patients undergoing immunotherapy may receive an adrenaline rinse before the allergen extract is administered, thus reducing the immune response to the administered allergen. Adrenaline is also used as a bronchodilator for asthma if specific β2 agonists are unavailable or ineffective.[7]

epipen (epinephrine autoinjector) is a medical device used to deliver a measured dose (or doses) of epinephrine (also known as adrenaline).An Epipen is used for the treatment of acute allergic reactions to avoid or treat the onset of anaphylactic shock.

granulocytes are a category of white blood cells characterized by the presence of granules in their cytoplasm.[1] There are three types of granulocytes,

granulocytes (con't) distinguished by their appearance under Wright's stain: neutrophils, eosinophils, and basophils.

histamine is an organic nitrogen compound involved in local immune responses as well as regulating physiological function in the gut and acting as a neurotransmitter.[2] Histamine triggers the inflammatory response. As part of an immune response to foreign pathogens, histamine is produced by basophils and by mast cells found in nearby connective tissues. Histamine increases the permeability of the capillaries to white blood cells and some proteins, to allow them to engage pathogens in the infected tissues.[3]

hypersensitivity (also called **hypersensitivity reaction** or **intolerance**) refers to undesirable reactions produced by the normal immune system, including allergies and autoimmunity. These reactions may be damaging, uncomfortable, or occasionally fatal. Hypersensitivity reactions require a pre-sensitized (immune) state of the host.

immunity is the state of having sufficient biological defenses to avoid infection, disease, or other unwanted biological invasion. It is the capability of the body to resist harmful microbes from entering it.

immunodeficiency (or **immune deficiency**) is a state in which the immune system's ability to fight infectious disease is compromised or entirely absent.

immunoglobulin E (IgE) is a class of antibody or immunoglobulin (Ig) "isotype" (related protein/genes) that's found only in mammals IgE also plays an essential role in type I hypersensitivity,[7] which manifests various allergic diseases, such as allergic asthma, allergic rhinitis,

immunoglobulin E (IgE con't) food allergy, and some types of chronic urticaria and atopic dermatitis. IgE plays a pivotal role, too, in allergic conditions, such as anaphylactic reactions to certain drugs, bee stings, and antigen preparations used in specific desensitization immunotherapy.

Immunoglobulin G (IgG) is an antibody isotype (related proteins/genes). Each IgG has two antigen binding sites. Antibodies are major components of the immune system. IgG is the main antibody isotype found in blood and extracellular fluid allowing it to control infection of body tissues. By binding many kinds of pathogens—representing viruses, bacteria, and fungi—IgG protects the body from infection. It does this via several immune mechanisms.

immunotherapy is a medical term defined as the "treatment of disease by inducing, enhancing, or suppressing an immune response".[1] Immunotherapies designed to elicit or amplify an immune response are classified as **activation immunotherapies,** while immunotherapies that reduce or suppress are classified as **suppression immunotherapies.**

isotype usually refers to any related proteins/genes from a particular gene family. In immunology, the "immunoglobulin isotype" refers to the genetic variations or differences in the constant regions of the heavy and light chains.

leukotrienes are a family of eicosanoid inflammatory mediators produced in leukocytes .[1][2] As their name leukotrienes implies, leukotrienes were first discovered in leukocytes, but have since been found in other immune cells. Leukotrienes use lipid signaling to convey information to either the cell producing them (autocrine

leukotrienes (con't) signaling or neighboring cells (paracrine signaling) in order to regulate immune responses. Leukotriene production is usually accompanied by the production of histamine and prostaglandins, which also act as inflammatory mediators. One of their roles (specifically, leukotriene D$_4$) is to trigger contractions in the smooth muscles lining the bronchioles; their overproduction is a major cause of inflammation in asthma and allergic rhinitis.[3] Leukotriene antagonists are used to treat these disorders by inhibiting the production or activity of leukotrienes.

lymphocyte is a kind of white blood cell in the vertebrate immune system,[1] specifically, a landmark of the adaptive immune system.Under the microscope, Lymphocytes can be divided into large lymphocytes and small lymphocytes. Large granular lymphocytes include natural killer cells (NK cells). Small lymphocytes consist of T cells and B cells.

lymphatic system is part of the circulatory system, comprising a network of conduits called lymphatic vessels that carry a clear fluid called lymph (from Latin *lympha* "water goddess"[1]) directionally towards the heart. The primary function of the lymph system is to provide an accessory route for these excess 3 litres per day to get returned to the blood.[2] Lymph is essentially recycled blood plasma. Lymphatic organs play an important part in the immune system, having a considerable overlap with the **lymphoid system.**

macrophages, (Greek: big eaters, from *makros* "large" + *phagein* "eat"), are cells produced by the differentiation of monocytes in tissues. Their role is to phagocytose, or engulf and then digest, cellular debris and pathogens, either as stationary or as mobile cells. They also stimulate lymphocytes and other immune cells to respond to

macrophages (con't) pathogens. They are specialized *phagocytic* cells that attack foreign substances, infectious microbes and cancer cells through destruction and ingestion. They are present in all living tissues, and have a function in regeneration.[3]

mast cell is a resident cell of several types of tissues and contains many granules rich in histamine and heparin. Although best known for their role in allergy and anaphylaxis, mast cells play an important protective role, as well, in being intimately involved in wound healing and defense against pathogens.[2] The mast cell is very similar in both appearance and function to the basophil, a type of white blood cell. However, they are not the same, as they arise from different cell lines.[3]

MAST CELL

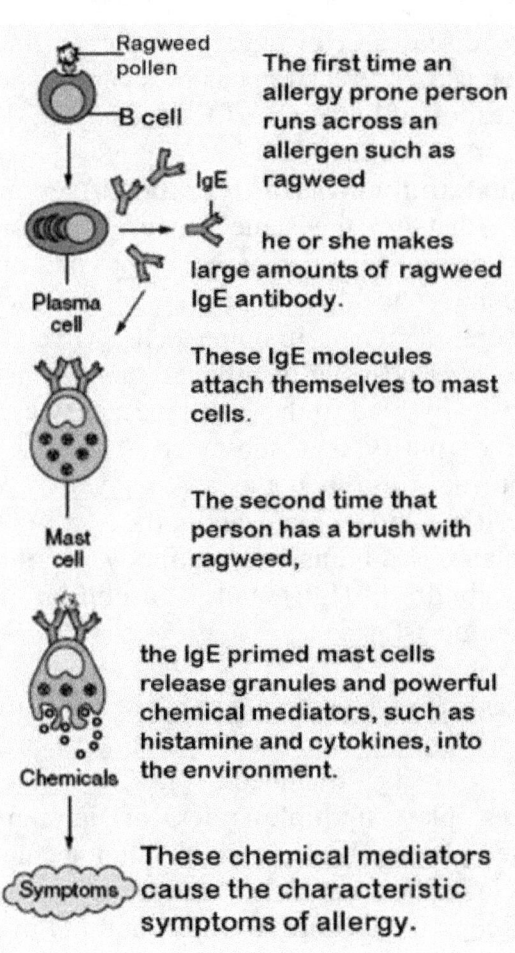

The first time an allergy prone person runs across an allergen such as ragweed

he or she makes large amounts of ragweed IgE antibody.

These IgE molecules attach themselves to mast cells.

The second time that person has a brush with ragweed,

the IgE primed mast cells release granules and powerful chemical mediators, such as histamine and cytokines, into the environment.

These chemical mediators cause the characteristic symptoms of allergy.

mistaken identity Allergic reactions occur when a person's immune system reacts to normally harmless substances. The hypersensitive person's body causes a false alarm reaction as it *"perceives"* a threat. Those who are **not** hypersensitive—mount significant Immunoglobulin E responses **only** as a defense against **real** threats, such as: infectious diseases. However, for allergic individuals, a trigger that causes a reaction can be a simple spec of dust or a tiny digestion of food. (Dr. J.K. Kansal, 9-6-13)

monoclonal antibodies (**mAb** or **moAb**) are monospecific antibodies that are the same because they are made by identical immune cells that are all clones of a unique parent cell, in contrast to polyclonal antibodies which are made from several different immune cells. Given almost any substance, it is possible to produce monoclonal antibodies that specifically bind to that substance; they can then serve to detect or purify that substance. This has become an important tool in biochemistry, molecular biology and medicine. One monoclonal antibody, Omalizumab (trade name Xolair), is a humanized antibody. It **inhibits** human immunoglobulin E (IgE) and is useful in moderate-to-severe allergic asthma.

monocytes are a type of white blood cell and are part of the innate immune system of vertebrates including all mammals (humans included), birds, reptiles, and fish. Monocytes play multiple roles in immune function. Monocytes play multiple roles in immune function. Such roles include: (1) replenish resident macrophages and dendritic cells under normal states, and (2) in response to inflammation signals, monocytes can move quickly (approx. 8–12 hours) to sites of infection in the tissues and divide/differentiate into macrophages and dendritic cells to elicit an immune response. Half of them are stored in the spleen.[1]

neutrophils are a type of phagocyte and are normally found in the blood stream. During the beginning (acute) phase of inflammation, particularly as a result of bacterial infection, environmental exposure,[4] and some cancers,[5][6] neutrophils are one of the first-responders of inflammatory cells to migrate towards the site of inflammation.. Neutrophils are recruited to the site of injury within minutes following trauma and are the hallmark of acute inflammation.[7]

pathogen (Greek: πάθος *pathos* "suffering, passion" and γενής *genēs* "producer of") in the oldest and broadest sense is anything that can produce disease.[1] Typically the term is used to mean an **infectious agent** (colloquially known as a *germ*) - a microorganism, in the widest sense such as a virus, bacterium, prion, or fungus, that causes disease in its host. The host may be an animal, human, a plant, or even another microorganism.

phagocytes are the cells that protect the body by ingesting (phagocytosing) harmful foreign particles, bacteria, and dead or dying cells. Their name comes from the Greek *phagein*, "to eat" or "devour", and "-cyte", the suffix in biology denoting "cell", from the Greek *kutos*, "hollow vessel".[1] They are essential for fighting infections and for subsequent immunity. The professional phagocytes include cells called: neutrophils, monocytes, macrophages, dendritic cells, and mast cells.[10]

proteins are large biological molecules consisting of one or more chains of amino acids. Proteins perform a vast array of functions within living organisms, including catalyzing metabolic reactions, replicating DNA, responding to stimuli, and transporting molecules from one location to another.

Samter's triad (It is named for Doctor Max Samter.) [21] Semester's triad is a medical condition consisting of asthma, aspirin and NSAID sensitivity, and nasal/ethmoidal polyposis.[1] It usually begins in young adulthood[2] (twenties and thirties are the most common onset times)[3] and may not include any other allergies. Initial reports on the link between asthma, aspirin and nasal polyposis were made by Widal in 1922.[22] Further studies were done by Samter & Beers in reports published in 1968.[23] It wasn't until 1968 when Samter and Beers described patients with the symptom triad of: asthma, aspirin sensitivity and nasal polyps that the condition became recognized and known as Samter's triad. Chronic hyperplastic sinusitis (enlargement caused by excessive multiplication of cells) is now considered a fourth hallmark of the disease, with the preferred name now being aspirin exacerbated respiratory disease (AERD).

T cells or **T lymphocytes** are a type of lymphocyte (itself a type of white blood cell) that play a central role in cell-mediated immunity. They are called T cells because they mature in the thymus.

White blood cells, or **leukocytes** (also spelled "leucocytes"), are cells of the immune system involved in defending the body against both infectious disease and foreign materials The name "white blood cell" derives from the fact that after centrifugation of a blood sample, the white cells are found in the *buffy coat*, a thin, typically white layer of nucleated cells between the sedimented red blood cells and the blood plasma. The scientific term *leukocyte* (from the Greek word *leuko-* meaning "white" and *kytos* meaning "hollow vessel", with -cyte translated as "cell" in modern usage) directly reflects this description.

.

MAIN CHARACTERS

ANTIBODIES:

Henry (Sergeant)
George (Sergeant)
Major Borline
Captain Kale
Sergeant Birlly
Private Richey
Private Porter
Corporeal Geno Getson (Vessel Patrol Officer)
Sergeant Deb Doss (Special Forces: Food Allergies)

ANTIGENS:

Vernie
Vance
Carlos
Tobie
Kristie
Kath
Gemly
Skidder
Karin and Ronnie (a couple of antibody converts)

The body, mind, spirit, and friendly, well-educated antibodies are the heroes. After all, if we are going to keep chasing life and cheating death as the wise doctor, Sanjay Gupta, advocates—we need that genuine holistic healthcare outlook.

Gail Galvan

CHAPTER 1

There's a war going on inside hypersensitive bodies between the antigens and us, the antibodies. Battlegrounds within bloodstreams, leaky fluids, cells, and body organs, a conglomeration of chemical reactions occur every minute. Sometimes we win, sometimes we lose, but my comrades and I always give it a good fight.

My name is Henry. I'm an antibody, a specialist in hypersensitivity. My enemies call me their worst enemy, someone to be wary of and avoid at all costs. You can think of me as an agent on a mission, a spy even, a good guy or a bad guy—because I can be both, as some of the following stories will attest to. (In military terms, I rank as a Sergeant.) Remember, though, I'm only one patriotic soldier in the war against allergies and immunological warfare, and I can merely tell you about the lives of a few of my buddies, but there are armies of us patrolling inside vulnerable human bodies. So don't think this is the whole story by any means.

Let's see, where should I begin, with the survivors or the casualties? This last case was the one that really turned my head around. I'll tell you about her. I've always been a sucker for high-spirited, cute 16 year old blondes. And this girl, Marin, had all it takes to make any creature's heart skip a beat. But a while ago, back in time, Marin "bit the dust," as the young kids say these days. What a heartbreaker. Her insatiable curiosity and zest for life was so impressive, her spirit so remarkable. She was special all right, and things will never be the same, not since Marin. Her death taught me everything I ever feared about the consequences of overreacting.

The day she died, a Saturday afternoon, lightning bolts kept flashing across the sky, but it wouldn't rain. Marin lived in a small Kansas town known for its vicious tornadoes. She told her mother that she was headed for the bowling alley with a couple of her friends. Mrs. McDonald urged her to be careful because of the oncoming storm. Of course Marin didn't like being treated like a little kid, so she wised off and gave her mom some static before she left.

"Mom, didn't I just have a birthday, you know, a year older, a year wiser? And haven't I always been real careful about any tornado warnings? When will you ever let me grow up? I love you Mom, but sometimes, you drive me nuts. You know J.J.'s has a shelter in case we need it, now I gotta go. Carrie's waiting for me."

"Okay, okay. Marin, go. I'll see you when you get home." By this time, Marin realized that she'd been a little too harsh on dear old Mom, so she tried to make up for it with a goodbye kiss.

"Bye Mom, I'll see you about five, okay?" She kissed her on the cheek and ran out the door.

Marin had been ill throughout her childhood and adolescence. She suffered from frequent episodes of hay fever, sinus problems, cold sores, asthma, and stomach aches. With age, the predicament worsened. Minor headaches became major ones. Her mild gastrointestinal upsets grew more serious, and included bouts of acute abdominal pain.

A family physician, troubled by the increased severity of symptoms, decided it was time to consult a specialist. Marin was finally referred to an allergist. The appointment was only a few days away. Now if the hometown doctor had known more about me, my enemies and pals, that we were actually at the root of her problems, much of Marin's suffering could have been alleviated, and her life saved.

Our power, as antibodies, to either protect or destroy is frequently underestimated. Often, people tend to blame emotional problems. Like Marin, sometimes her mom and the doctor believed the complaints were a teenager's way of rebelling and gaining attention, or a method of playing

2

hooky from school. Of course, the mind and body are both important to consider, but for people, even experts in the field of psychology, to deny my existence with so much obvious proof. Wise up. Especially these days, we're busier than ever fighting off environmental stressors that hypersensitive people can't seem to adapt to.

I understand what some psychologists believe. The mind can be so influential in causing or combating disease. But so often, it's the misunderstanding and lack of proper education and health care that causes an unnecessary death of an allergic or asthmatic victim. Just like Marin, all she needed was a lifesaver kit, one shot of epinephrine and she might have made it to the hospital. Now all we can do is hopefully learn from our mistakes.

Anyway, Marin had allergies, severe ones. It was one of those cases where nobody paid any attention to them, me or my pals. I tried to pull out at the last minute when I realized it was too late, but the damage was done. It happened right on the floor of the bowling alley. A yellow jacket was the culprit. Don't ask me how it got inside, but there it flew, buzzing around as if it owned the place. Everyone began to squirm around, giggling and screaming like typical teenage girls, except for Marin. She wanted to take care of the problem so that the bowling could continue.

"You guys, it's just a dumb old bee. I'm gonna get a shoe and kill it. Carrie, give me your tennis shoe." Carrie reached under the seating area and looked for her shoe, but couldn't find it, so she tossed a sandal to Marin.

"Here. Be careful."

"There he is over on that chair! God, he's big. Oh, be careful, Marin, if you miss I hear they really get mad and come after you." One of the girls pointed and backed up.

"Okay. Here goes." She tiptoed over toward the yellow jacket and slammed the shoe down to squash it.

"Oh shoot, watch out I missed him. Stupid bee, moved right at the last minute. There he is. Watch out Patti!" By this time the girls and several others were yelling and shuffling around, so the man at the front desk ran over and asked what the commotion was.

"I'm trying to kill this darn bee. Do you have a fly swatter? Maybe we could kill it that way," Marin said.

"Marin, watch out, there he is on your back. Get him off, somebody!" Carrie yelled as she ran toward her.

"OW! He stung me, get him off!" Marin screamed while swinging her arms.

"There, I got him," Carrie said as she stomped on the bee after it had fallen to the floor. "Come over here. Are you all right?" Her friends followed Marin as she went to sit down.

"Yeah, I guess I'm okay. That hurt though. Did you get the stupid bee? We should have just left him alone." She raised her shirt and asked Carrie to take a look at it. "Is it red, Carrie, or what?"

"Yes, it's red all right and it looks like it's swelling too. We better get you home."

But Marin never made it home. She never even made it to the door. The villain had struck an innocent victim. I guess bees do their good in the world too, and it's really the over-zealous antibodies who are the true enemies, but to allergic victims, believe me, bees can be killers, even if it is indirectly.

Anyway, at the point of impact, it was our duty to step in and try to battle the poison. We were ready. My friends and I were always ready. That was the problem, we liked to fight, and we got so we did it too often and too viciously. Our intentions were good, but it didn't matter. Her immune system got out of hand and the poor kid died. Anaphylactic shock. She started breathing funny and I could actually see her muscle fibers tightening up. I told everyone to pull back, that we were fighting the antigens too much. But

4

everything had gone haywire and I knew it was too late. She became unconscious and the next thing to go was her heart. What a scene, a sad story. She died, like I said, right there on the bowling alley floor.

You can see how terrible I feel. Here I am a do-gooder gone sour. Not that I haven't done my share of saving lives and helping people fight their allergies.

Believe me, the life of an antibody soldier isn't the easiest, most flamboyant job in the world. But we lost her, and it certainly took its toll on me that day. So I decided to spill my guts, tell you the inside story, the nitty gritty about those creeps, the allergies.

Now if you're at all familiar with the life cycle of an antibody, you probably won't believe a word of any of this. Don't ask me why I'm still around, assigned to case after case. I lost many of my buddies when Marin died. I thought that's the way it worked, when the host dies, so do I. Maybe I'm destined to live out one scenario after another, until I get it right or until I've learned all I'm supposed to, I don't know. Maybe it's reincarnation. But if it is, I remember all of my past cases.

So if I tell you my story, what's in it for me? Well everything. Sometimes in a lifetime—animals, human beings, even fourth world creatures, as we're sometimes called; we all feel as if there is something we must do. Well, it's my turn. I've got to do it for Marin, for me, because if I don't, allergies will go on destroying people, and it's not fair, because they're really the bad guys, not us, the antibodies.

CHAPTER 2

Death isn't always the end result from an allergy attack. Marin's was certainly one of the most unfortunate cases I can recall. But believe me, allergies are permeating people's lives and causing a great deal of subtle, as well as obvious and profound physical and mental distress. They have got to be stopped.

I remember one young couple who lived in Akron, Ohio. Tim and Barb knew the essence of love, at least for the first few years anyway. Oh, everyone knew that sooner or later they'd be forced to come down to Earth with their ideal love. But, I know the inside story and one of the main causes of their marital deterioration. Barb endured significant allergies which constantly toyed with her body and caused all sorts of reactions. We fought them for years, but could not get rid of them. She experienced an assortment of adverse effects, from ugly cold sores, itchy red eyes, nausea and ulcer-like symptoms, to painful migraines and an increasingly despondent nature. She began to lose her pizzazz and consequently, Tim began to lose interest. One night they had a big fight.

"Go to the New Year's party without me. I don't care, I don't feel good anyway," Barb said sarcastically.

"That's the problem, you never feel good. I'm sorry, but I'm tired of hearing about it. And we can't afford any more of those tests. We're running out of money just because you never feel well. And I can't sit around and babysit you, because I want to live a happy life. Do you know what that means, a happy life? Remember when we were happy?" Tim hurried toward the front door.

Of course Barb burst into tears. "Go out and have fun. You deserve it." She wiped the tears from her eyes.

"But so do I, and it's not fair. It's not my fault that I'm sick again. I'm trying as hard as I can." She walked over to the sink in the kitchen to get a glass of water and a tissue or paper towel to blow her nose. "That's all, just go. Oh, I hate it, I hate it. I hate being sick!" She cried uncontrollably and hit her fist on the table as she sat back down.

"You're just getting to be a nagging neurotic, that's all there is to it. I'm sorry sweetheart, but I'm not letting your problems spoil my New Years. Now if you want to get dressed, we'll go together, otherwise I'm leaving right now." He looked directly at her and awaited an answer.

"Go. Just go. I can't. I feel terrible." So he left and slammed the door behind him. Afterward, Barb took two aspirins, two tablespoons of Pepto Bismol, turned the radio on, climbed into bed feeling alienated, guilty and hurt, and cried herself to sleep.

The friction kept worsening between the two "lovebirds" because of Barb's poor health, and their marriage began to crumble. However, fortunately in this case, Barb's doctor soon recommended a specialist, an internist, who in turn referred her to an allergist. After a comprehensive physical and mental examination, some scrutinizing of her medical history and allergy tests, the doctor concluded that Barb definitely had some allergy related medical problems. They were so thrilled to finally have some answers.

Within three months time, she was aware of many of the causes of her illness. The couple moved from the damp, moldy basement apartment which they had been living in, and obtained the help of a qualified nutritionist. Barb stopped taking aspirin and an oral contraceptive which she found had caused some of her reactions. In time she began an exercise program and gradually began to feel healthier. After a while, she lost the nervousness and fatigue which had accompanied her debilitated condition. Barb and Tim soon found their love for each other and marriage to be happily intact once again.

That's one inspiring story about a marriage that survived an allergy affliction. Unfortunately, thousands of others have failed under similar circumstances, not solely because someone in the family had an allergy, but in many cases, partly because of it. Allergies create stress, and stress creates allergies. Those allergy creeps like to take advantage of bodies with lowered resistance. On the other hand, so many times they're responsible for lowering the resistance, (or heightening immune system reactions, I should say), especially when an individual can't manage to obtain adequate rest. So there you have it, the vicious cycle.

CHAPTER 3

Swelling is one of the reactions that allergies like to cause and it's something they do very well. Once they attack, we try to fight back; then a chemical called histamine is released and swelling occurs.

One of the worst places for this phenomenon to take place is within the hearing apparatus. It happened one time to Kevin, a little boy I liked. There is another sad truth to this story. I was partially to blame for causing Kevin's deafness.

Only five at the time, he was a very amiable little guy. His mom came home from the allergist's office one day, with the, luckily, not so bad news. She would not have known how to break it to her husband or Kevin if the answer was no again, the deafness irreparable. The allergist had finally found a surgeon who could help. Eventually Kevin would be able to hear again.

Mrs. Koleski sat down at the dinner table one night and explained what the doctor told her. "Dr. Bates says that Kevin's hearing loss is correctable. Thank God. We'll continue to treat this latest infection, but as soon as it clears up we can try the surgery. He assured me that it's going to be okay. You're going to be all right Kevin." She stood up and walked over to her son, hugged him, and then made the appropriate gestures to help him understand what she was saying. Kevin said the first thing he wanted to hear again was his cartoons. The three of them cried and hugged each other. Later that evening, Mr. and Mrs. Koleski sat up in bed talking to each other, expressing both guilt and relief.

"Why? How did we let him get this bad? Why didn't we get to the cause of it sooner? Why?" questioned Mrs. Koleski.

"I don't know dear, that's a very good question." He looked up toward the ceiling; then leaned his head over on his wife's shoulder. "I don't know why. We just kept thinking he would get better. Kev doesn't deserve this. We've learned our lesson. From now on, we take his allergies very seriously. We'll watch him really close. Okay honey? He's going to be all right." They embraced. Within minutes they were both asleep. Tomorrow they could begin to move away from their nightmare.

Shortly before six, the alarm clock beeped loudly. After realizing their good fortune, the beauty of something called a "second chance," the Koleskis both stared at each other and smiled. The sun glistened through the silk curtains and a cool, soft breeze swept across their faces. But the sound emitting from the television in the living room reminded them, too quickly, that their deaf son sat watching the early morning cartoons unable to hear the animated voices of Bugs Bunny and the Smurfs. He'll hear them again soon. Thank God, just a little longer, Kev, they both thought to themselves.

Do you see how it works? Allergies are the antagonists. We just try to counterattack. Trouble is, there is a fine line between protecting and maintaining an equilibrium within the human body and the other extreme of causing an all out war, a hyper-reaction.

CHAPTER 4

It's remarkable what the human body can tolerate. I've been involved with the heavy drinkers, modern-day pot heads, cocaine sniffers, food addicts, smokers, and the caffeine and sugar extremists. And every time I enter into a specific case, I say to myself, "Don't you know there's a war going on inside here? Have some mercy! Give us a break!" Things begin to break down or spin out of control, and no antibody in the world should be subjected to the kind of torture or workload people throw at us.

The sad part is that they don't know how lucky they are. If they'd just wise up and think about how important there health is. But then, who am I to judge humans? I know they have their "grounds of existence," just like we do. Like all of the black lung or asbestosis cases. Maybe sometimes, socio-economic reasons make it necessary that some people work certain jobs which cause these deadly diseases. But when it's a matter of life and breath, all I keep thinking about is that there's got to be another way. There's just got to.

It's sad enough when the innocent victims get sick, but the self-destructive ones who have a choice and take part in digging their own premature graves, those cases simply flabbergast me. You'd think that by now, Americans, the French, Germans, Italians, Russians, Asians, Indians, Mexicans, all different cultures and species would possess some sophisticated, sound, basic knowledge about their bodies and minds in regards to feeling healthy.

Then there's the other side of the coin, too, the one that drives me half crazy. That's the "supplemented" generation. I'm referring to the individual who can't stop thinking about health. With adequate health education, seems like it should happen naturally, easily, if people follow basic principles. Not so much an obsession. I suppose everyone has to find their own way and I don't discredit anyone's willingness and desire to search. Sometimes, though, I just feel like there is too much talk and not enough proper action. After Eastern philosophies, nutrition fads and a multitude of various supplements and ideologies to escape the responsibility of coming right back to where people started, namely themselves; where does the individual go then? That's my question.

It's the ones making a sincere effort to get well or remain healthy that I care about. People like Marin, Barb, the Koleskis and Captain Ramon Rodz, a navy pilot who needed my help for a while.

We flew over deserts, oceans, wastelands, mountains, vast prairies, countries and all over the United States. He knew how to handle a plane the way a Pope guides a congregation through a prayer—smoothly, serenely, and with never-ending courage and reassurance. Captain Rodz was the best. I'm not going to elaborate here on another case of mine gone haywire, so don't worry. On the contrary, the Captain had everything under control and his life was something to marvel at. I think he even slept with a good sense of humor and purpose in mind.

But he wasn't immune to occasional problems, and one particular thing was beginning to annoy him. For about the last month, every time he flew, approximately an hour or so after takeoff, he started sneezing. He experienced tightness in his chest, itched, felt lethargic and nauseous and also suffered from mild visual blurring and an annoying ringing in his ears.

Since Captain Rodz was well aware of all the lives he was responsible for, as he readied for takeoff one day, he vowed to himself that he would not fly again until the cause for his disconcerting symptoms was discovered. Fortunately, his family physician suspected an allergy and referred him to an allergist, so it didn't take long to find the culprit.

"First, Captain, let me assure you that your physical exam results were fine, nothing out of the ordinary or any medical issues showed up. But that's common in cases like this. I realize however, that you do have some type of unique problem that could be very dangerous in your line of work. Now I'm going to ask you to try to be specific as I ask you some questions," the doctor explained.

"Go right ahead Doctor, that's why I'm here. I'll do my best." He crossed his legs and leaned back in the chair.

"Okay. I want you to tell me if you can think of any strong odors which you are aware of each time you enter the plane or cockpit. Can you think of any scents which stand out?" he asked.

"Well, let's see, I never really thought about it. I think a few of the flight attendants wear perfume, but nothing very distinguishable. And I do smell a certain type of cleansing agent, occasionally, on the instrument board. But, it doesn't seem to bother me. Other than that, I can't really think of anything."

"That's good, exactly the type of things I need to know. Now, tell me what you usually eat the night before a flight. I'm especially looking for a favorite food or one that you eat regularly before each flight."

The captain began to laugh, but then regained his serious, cooperative self. "Oh Lord, what do I eat? It varies so much. My wife, Sherry, makes a delicious lasagna dinner on certain nights when I'm home," Captain Rodz answered.

Dr. Wilson uncrossed his arms and smiled. He sat in a brown leather chair and leaned forward with a pen in his hand ready to write down everything mentioned.

"I'll tell you Doctor, my main dinners in the evening usually consist of chicken, fish occasionally, usually perch, a good T-bone steak and some Italian or Mexican food. In Phoenix, Arizona I have a favorite Chinese restaurant, usually it's chicken and broccoli. My other favorite

13

vegetables are corn, fried okra and cauliflower with cheese sauce and salads. I do eat a lot of salads with vinegar and oil. I don't eat shrimp because of a severe reaction once."

"Very good. Now, can you think of anything else?" asked Dr. Wilson.

"I think that's about it."

The phone rang and interrupted their detective work for a few minutes. Then the doctor persisted and wanted to know about desserts, beverages and breakfast selections.

"Oh, for desserts, let's see, that would be cheesecake, Sherry's homemade apple cobbler, or vanilla ice cream or orange sherbet when I'm on the road. For breakfast, that's simple, scrambled eggs, bacon, toast, a glass of orange juice and plenty of black coffee."

"How much coffee do you drink?"

"Usually about three cups, but I switched to decaffeinated a while back because I was getting some headaches." After a short pause, Captain Rodz continued to disclose more dietary information. "And I do drink a couple beers occasionally or some ice tea or water."

"Do you drink much milk or pop?" asked Dr. Wilson.

"No, I never cared that much for either." He shook his head no.

"Okay, now, can you think of anything else, particularly anything unusual you've been eating lately, something you don't ordinarily..."

The Captain interrupted. "Wait a minute, there is something I've been eating lately that I don't usually eat, for the last month or so. Doctor, I think you're a genius. Is it possible to have the kind of symptoms I've been having from eating a lot of walnuts?"

"It's possible, Captain. Some people do have specific serious allergies to peanuts or walnuts." Both men smiled and realized that they had probably just finished their little game of Sherlock Holmes and Dr. Watson. "Are you eating them prior to flying or the night before or what?" asked the Doctor.

"Let me tell you how I got hooked on them. Peggy, a new neighbor from next door, apparently buys a bulk quantity of nuts wholesale each month and then ends up selling them. My wife has been buying walnuts and peanuts and stuffing them in my pockets and suitcase before I leave home. And, I keep eating more and more each flight. I've gotten used to them, is that it Doctor?"

The Captain asked inquisitively.

"Well, we won't know for sure until we administer some tests, but it certainly sounds possible. I'd like you to go down to the second floor, to the allergy testing lab and ask for Dr. Teller, and we'll find out. He's waiting for you. I told him you'd be down sometime this afternoon. They'll also pull your chart and take a good look at it. In the meantime, don't eat any more nuts. I think we might be getting there." He stood up and offered to shake the Captain's hand.

They shook hands and exchanged smiles as Captain Rodz thanked the doctor, then turned to walk out the door.

"Now, they'll fill you in on all of the details downstairs. We'll follow up on this after all your tests." said Dr. Wilson.

They had figured it out. As soon as the Captain refrained from eating the daily walnuts, the physical symptoms (which had become such a nuisance and potential occupational and health hazard) subsided and finally disappeared.

A word of caution, here, if I might. What the Doctor said is true, some people have food allergies. But this is another controversial matter which drives me half crazy. On one hand, there are people out there with legitimate food allergies or intolerances. Many allergic victims suffer for years because the cause of their disruptive bodily reactions cannot be detected. Then there are actually children and/or adults starving or panicking at the sight of anything edible, because they have been frightened into believing that they are allergic to everything. In other words, to survive, the individual would actually be forced to live in a protective shield of some sort and avoid food, the enemy.

Dr. Coballan, a specialist in food allergies, cautions people to determine legitimate food reactions in an objective way, not to overreact, and remember how important nutrition can be to health. He wrote a book on the subject.

I learned a lot from him and some other doctors about the good old "mistaken identity" phenomenon—how "perceived" threats are causing much of the chaos within the hypersensitive bodies we're trying to get under control. I tell them, "Yeah, we still have to fight off the bad guys, infectious agents and true harmful enemies, but, again, so many of the antibody troops won't listen. Not sure what I can do to get them to stop reacting to false alarms. All I know is they need to back off before more people get hurt.

CHAPTER 5

As I said before, I've been around, and one of the places where I've spent a lot of time is in the school classroom. From the west coast to the east, up to Canada, throughout the Midwestern and southern states, into Europe, and all around the globe, antibodies are prevalent residents. Allergy is a common cause of infancy and childhood disorders. What bothers me about the area of disease is the fact that despite all of our endeavors to make it clear that allergies are the antagonists, so often, nobody pays attention.

Consequently, allergies and asthma frequently become two of the most unattended and devastating developmentally disabling diseases known to the human race. The magnitude of the damage to the human spirit and potential resulting from allergic and asthmatic diseases may never be fully realized. Not only physical damage, but some emotional or sociological damage can result as well, partially because any disease affects all facets of a person's life. Allergies and asthma, and all of the debilitating side effects which accompany these diseases, are quite often not obvious to human eyesight or perceptible, the way other handicaps might be. But these diseases cause havoc just the way other afflictions do.

Yet the asthmatic or allergic sufferer is grateful for the reversible nature of symptoms and the healthy days experienced, the days or hours when, although vulnerable, they can still enjoy life in a healthy way.

Statistics? If you really want to hear the facts, I've got lots of figures. I'm talking millions of afflicted people, and millions of lost days from school, work and life in general. I could go on and on, all of the interesting people I've known, humans from all walks of life, including celebrities, brilliant inventors, artists, and musicians, the athletes. I even tried to help a President once, but his medical friends never seemed to make the connection and failed to get to the source of the problem, even after all the alarms we set off. He suffered so needlessly. I'd like to talk about that case, but I'm afraid I'm due on another one, a follow-up, someone I've known for a long time, but left on her own a few years back, because she didn't need me anymore.

I want to see how Sara's doing, see if she finally resolved everything. She wrote about her life too, a book called *Gone with the Tires*, in which she tells about her bicycle touring trip along the Pacific Coast. It meant a lot to her because she was an asthmatic who had struggled with allergies all her life. I suppose it was Sara's turning point.

Can this actually be the girl I used to know? She looks healthier than ever. Her journeys through life and health education studies must have paid off. But, I always knew she was a fighter, that's why I left earlier than usual. She was making all the right moves, so I figured she'd obtain quality health sooner or later.

It looks like she's on vacation, at home with her relatives in Indiana. Everything looks good, this could be fun. It'll be nice to be back in the swing of live action again, and not pulling everything from memory. Besides,

I could use a vacation and some fun myself, as long as I'm getting my point across.

CHAPTER 6

"Toss me a cigarette, Stacy, and your lighter," Sara requested. The two young women sat across from each other at a dining room table.

"No. My sister does not smoke," Stacy professed as she grabbed the package of Marlboro Lights and held onto them tightly.

"C'mon. I'm tired of being different. I won't inhale, it's just my way of adapting, relaxing and not letting the smoke get to my head or my lungs." The two of them wrestled until Sara managed to free the package of cigarettes from Stacy's hands. "I know as long as I'm visiting, I'd better get used to the smoke."

"No!" Stacy persisted.

"Yes! I just want to have one, okay." Sara put the cigarette in her mouth and lit it, began to puff on it and emit smoke into the air. "See, no big deal." Stacy started to laugh and shook her head in disbelief.

"You've changed."

"Why, what do you mean?" Sara smiled.

"I don't think you should be smoking. That's not you at all. It used to be all you'd do is come back here and complain about it to Mom or Dad or me." Stacy looked surprised again as Sara took another puff.

"I know, huh. Well, I'll tell you something Stacy. It took me a lot of years to learn how to be healthy because of that dumb asthma and my allergies. But once I did gain my health, I kept on going and going until I felt as if I had reached a point where nothing could hurt me, if I didn't let it. But I did find out the hard once, when I ran out of my inhaler, and had no back up around, just how dangerous it is to be careless when two puffs can save my life. Finally, Sara took two quick puffs and put the cigarette out.

"Well, I'd really rather see you taking puffs from an inhaler than puffs off a cigarette, that's for sure! Stacy laughed, stood up and walked away from the kitchen table to see what her young son Tommy wanted.

"Mom, can I play over at Holly's on the swing set?"

"Is Holly home?" Stacy asked as she bent down to tie Tommy's tennis shoe.

"Yeah. She's right there," he pointed, "in the front yard."

"Okay, but where's your sister? Is she still next door?"

"Yeah, she is. Bye." He ran out the door. Stacy walked to the refrigerator and opened the door to the freezing compartment. She dropped ice cubes into the green Tupperware glasses and filled them to the top with pink lemonade.

"Bye Tommy," Sara yelled from the front doorway. "Stacy, I'll turn the music back on. Let's listen to that one song again. What time's Hank coming home?"

"I think about five. He went to see about his job that starts tomorrow. So are you going up to Mom and Dad's later?" She handed a glass to Sara as they both sat down.

"Thanks. Yeah, I think I will. I was having fun the other night playing bartender and pool. I was winning at pool. I have to go get my quarters from my shorts, for the jukebox. Do you guys want to come tonight? Any possibility that Hank's mom and dad would babysit?"

"No! They sure won't if they know we're going to the bar. They take 'em on Saturday nights, though, so maybe we can go then."

"Okay, sounds good. Oh no, look at the time, I better get ready to go. I want to catch Dad before he leaves." She walked toward the bedroom, almost tripped over the toy collie that scratched vigorously in the hallway. Sara stopped momentarily to comb her hair in the bathroom.

"Hey Stacy, have you seen my yellow shorts? They aren't where I left them!" She shouted from the bedroom doorway.

"Oh, um," she paused, "try under the bed, the kids were playing in there this morning."

"All right," Sara lifted the disheveled covers from the bed and shook them to see if the shorts were intermingled between the sheet and the bedspread, then looked under the bed to no avail. She grabbed the bedpost and slid the bed to the left slightly and heard the quarters jingling. "There you are," she said and unsnapped the two pockets on the right and transferred a handful of quarters from her shorts to her jacket pocket.

"Stacy, listen," Sara walked toward the kitchen, "if Dave should call, tell him I'll be at Mom's in the morning so he can call over there, okay. We're supposed to go sailing tomorrow."

"Oh, you're gonna stay at Mom and Dad's tonight?"

"Yeah, I think so, rather than driving all the way back over here."

"Okay, I'll tell him." She moved toward Sara to give her a hug.

"Achoo! Oh my stupid nose." Sara reached for the paper towels on a counter top to the left.

"What's the matter?"

"Oh you know, it's my sneezing season again. My nose and eyes have been acting up since last week. Had to take an antihistamine this morning and I was okay for a while, but now it's acting up again. I hate to take them because they make me sleepy," Sara sniffled.

"I heard on the news today that it's the height of the hay fever season. Hank's been having trouble too."

"Sure is. Guess I'll have to survive it as usual though, that's all. How's his asthma been lately?"

While Sara inched her way toward the front door after making sure she had her purse, Stacy explained that Hank was much better since he left his job at the chemical plant.

"Well listen Stacy, I'd better get going. It is so good to see you and talk with you again. God I miss everyone so much. You know we have the neatest, most loving family there is. I may just have to move back here in a couple of years. The thing is, Colorado feels like home too. I'm always split between two homes, here and there. I sure am healthier there though, with the dry climate, you know."

"I know Sara, but we miss you a lot and it is nice to have you around." Stacy smiled.

"Well, we'll see. Then I'll see you tomorrow evening sometime, right?" She gave Stacy a hug.

"Sure. That'll be great. See ya later, and have fun." As Sara walked out the front door, she smiled back at her sister, then several children began to say hello and ask if they could go for a ride in her truck. "Well, sorry, "I have to go somewhere right now, but maybe tomorrow, okay?"

Later at the bar, Sara sat on a barstool and listened to some loud country-western tunes that played on the jukebox, while she talked to her dad.

"I saw Laura and Bill today, and their five kids. She lives in a beautiful house out in Chesterton, and she has a forest for a front and back yard. Really Dad, it's a nice old country-type house and her kids are so neat." Sara glanced toward the pool table and then quickly turned her head back toward her father.

"Oh. That's great. Laura. Do I know her? Oh, now I remember, the one with the long hair, your friend from high school," he said as he turned to ask the couple at the end of the bar if they would like another beer. "Just a second." He walked around the corner where the beer was stocked and got out two Old Styles, opened them quickly, set them down in front of the two customers, and then rang up two dollars on the cash register.

He walked back to Sara. "So they live in Chesterton? What road is that off of, if the house is located in the country?"

"You just exit the toll road off of Route 49, about three fourths of a mile turn left on the road before the viaduct and they're right down the street, but they're hidden behind a bunch of trees," explained Sara.

"Hmm. It sounds nice. I think I know that area. So you've been visiting everyone and having a good time, huh? Have you seen Dave? When are you two gonna get back together?" Her father asked. "I know you still love each other."

"We're supposed to go sailing tomorrow," replied Sara. "Dad, we're friends, and I'll always love him, that's all I can say. Everything has just changed so much, what we had is in the past." She turned and looked to see who walked in the door.

"Hi Mitch, how are ya?" Sara's dad headed back to the end of the bar again to get Mitch his usual to drink.

A red-haired lady sat at the other end of the bar and remarked, "There he is, Mitch the Magic Man." She turned toward the man who sat next to her, "This guy is good, honey, watch what he can do. Mitch, do the cigarette trick."

"I'm not doin' any tricks until I get me a cold beer, then I shall perform. John, where's my beer at?" The young man with wavy brown hair asked.

"Sure Mitch, here it is." John set the Miller's down, then rang it up.

"Hey, I know that guy," said a gray-haired, middle-aged man in a blue overall suit, standing at the bar. "He's the one who got his belly button cut off in Vietnam." A burst of laughter sounded throughout the bar, following the remark.

"You have a rowdy crowd in here sometimes, don't you?" Sara whispered to her father as she leaned toward him.

"Yes, we do, we really do." he nodded. "Listen Sara, your mother should be here any second, and Julie to take my place. We're going out to dinner. You're coming along, aren't you?"

"Sure. That's why I'm here, to spend time with you guys."

"Well that's what we'll do as soon as she gets here."

"Great Dad," Sara reached into her pocket for a few more quarters because the music had stopped, and she wanted to liven up the place again.

Now see, this is what I don't like about this job. Just when I start having fun or getting to like the people I'm around, I'm expected to drop everything and I'm required to jump right into a more challenging and less leisurely situation. At least I know that things worked out pretty good for Sara. When I think about how she almost died so many times, or how easily she could have ended up on an oxygen tank, or sneezing and wheezing her life away, because of her asthma and allergies. But she's not; she's got the control now. It makes me feel proud. Oh well, when duty calls. Another emergency I guess.

CHAPTER 7

Where am I anyway? What is this place? Let me look at my orders. I'm stationed back in Denver now. Several people are lounging in beige, cushioned chairs, scanning magazines. I'm watching two young children play with bright-colored toys in the corner, and one woman is just staring into space. A small-framed man, confined to a wheelchair with tubing in his nose and an oxygen tank at his side, just told a joke to his wife and a nurse.

The nurse tried to look interested, but obviously, she has other things on her mind. She laughed at the punch line and then excused herself, picked up a chart from a basket on the receptionist's desk and walked into a square-shaped room. Another nurse listened carefully as she took a patient's blood pressure.

"Mrs. Beller, we just need to get one more thing now. You know how to do this, right?" The nurse reached to assist the patient.

"Oh yes," she said as she stood up slowly, holding onto the nurse's shoulder. "I've done it plenty of times. Just let me catch my breath first. I had a rough night last night with my attack."

"Okay, you just take your time, whenever you're ready. Stand right up here, just a little closer, and I'll put a chair behind you."

"Right here?" Mrs. Beller asked. As she tried to catch her breath, wheezing sounds became audible.

"You are having a rough time today, aren't you? Yes, that's fine. Now, let me put this in here and hand this to you whenever you're ready. Remember, blow as hard and as long as you can," explained the nurse.

"All right," agreed Mrs. Beller. She placed the circular-shaped cardboard mouthpiece into her mouth, took a deep breath, held her hand on her chest and exhaled into the device.

"And blow, blow, blow, keep going, keep going. Good, a little longer. Good, that's it!" the nurse said enthusiastically. The patient's face reddened while she coughed harshly. The nurse cautiously watched Mrs. Beller and offered her a Kleenex.

"Here. Are you all right now? Just relax a minute. You know it makes people cough like that."

"Oh I'm fine now. It's just for a little bit, I just can't help it, it makes me cough." Mrs. Beller blew her nose again.

"Now, let me see if Dr. Loy is ready to see you. I'll be right back." The nurse walked down a hallway, wrote something next to Mrs. Beller's name on a piece of paper, wrote the patient's name and the doctor's name on an erasable schedule board, and then returned to the work-up room where the patient sat waiting.

"Okay, Mrs. Beller, follow me, right down here to room four and Dr. Loy will be right in." They walked toward the room. The nurse put Mrs. Beller's chart in a holder outside the door on the wall.

"Just have a seat, and he'll be right in," she smiled.

"All right, thank you." Mrs. Beller laid her purse down next to the chair.

Well, I figured out where I am. It's obvious that I'm in an allergy/respiratory clinic of some sort. Look at these charts, sinus infections, asthma, food sensitivities, allergies, immune diseases, and those people out there, now it's really getting crowded with patients looking for some relief. The anguish on their faces, the tissues in their hands, and the familiar mature attitude of acceptance, even from the kids. I've seen it all so many times before. At least these days there are clinics like this one to rehabilitate them, give them hope and a way to work toward a healthier existence.

This assignment is unusual for me. I'm usually on a one to one basis, but there are allergic and asthmatic sufferers all over this place that could use my assistance. Evidently I'm here as an observer, because I'm inside this one nurse, not a patient. That's fine with me. The work that needs to be done here looks overwhelming anyway.

But I'm sure I'm here for some important reason. Something is in store for me; I'd make a fifty dollar bet on that. I think I'll head up toward the blood lines and see if any of my old buddies are anywhere in the near vicinity.

CHAPTER 8

"Our duty, our mission, will remain the same: to serve, protect and preserve mankind through advanced biomedical endeavors in the areas of immunological medicine. You have played an essential role in providing information on immune-deficiency, allergic and autoimmune diseases. Above all, tonight, you are saluted for your devotion toward humanitarian goals." As the speech ended, the high-ranking antibody stepped down from the diaphragmatic stage, the crowd dispersed, and everyone headed back to their plasmic living quarters.

"George, is that you?" I asked.

"Henry, my God, you son of a gun, what the heck are you doing here?" George asked. We exchanged affectionate grins.

"Just got here, you know how the top brass works, right smack dab in the middle of some fun, back in the Midwest, and the next thing I know, my papers are in and here I am. What's the situation look like anyway? Well, never mind for now, you can tell me later. Tell me how life's been treating you."

"Oh, things are pretty good. Can't complain. My luck's been all right, not too many sad cases, some aspirin allergy cases, but most of them have been real promising with desensitization. Just got off of one of those adolescent cases, you know how they can go downhill fast, if someone doesn't work with 'em. J.D. had the works: allergies, asthma, emotional problems, learning difficulties, a doomed to fail attitude. You name it, he had it all. But that young man shaped up so fast once he enrolled in a school for learning disabled kids. He started trusting his teachers and realized they weren't trying to take his individuality away, only give him a chance, so he could start getting some education. Of course, the saddest case I had was a thirty-six year old woman with the big one, AIDS. Not sure why I was there, I couldn't be effective. Nothing worked. She hung in there for years, but then she died. So anyway, how about you? What's this about the Midwest?" George looked at me with his usual curious manner.

"Oh, had to go see about a follow-up. Remember Sara, the one with all the allergies and asthma when she was growing up, back in the Fifties and Sixties? The one allergic to aspirin, watermelon but she ate it anyway and her mom and dad smoked?"

"Sure I remember Sara, loved to run but always had trouble in gym class and used to take us to the movies all the time, had the hay fever in the summer, cold sores and asthma attacks. You sure did spend a lot of time with that girl. How's it looking for her nowadays, okay?" George asked.

"Well, all right for the most part, but do you know what that character was doing? Smoking!"

"Smoking? That's impossible, the way she used to yell at her mom and dad and brother. Are you kidding me?"

(I knew George would not believe it.) "I'm not fooling you. She only smoked one time at her sister's house, but she was definitely smoking. Said she wouldn't inhale, but she was tired of being different, and it was her way of letting go of the fear of cigarette smoke. Explained she felt so well, nothing could bother her anymore."

"Well," remarked George, "maybe she was just trying to prove a point or something." He paused.

"Could be, thing is, I know her. She's got a dog, you know, and sometimes she thinks she can just deny her potentially allergic condition, and then she gets run down and the asthma flares up," I explained.

"Know what you mean, it happens all the time, but you know what, I'd rather see her react that way. This is my own personal opinion now, but I'd rather see her do that than act like she's afraid of everything. Remember that one family, the Roberts and how they sold their little boy's bike because he had asthma. His grandfather tried to tell them to keep it, but they sold it and the boy kept failing after that, anything new he'd try, he just kept deteriorating, and got weaker every day. Had to spend so much time alone because the other kids didn't want to play with him. You see my point?" asked George.

I nodded and concluded in agreement that Sara possibly knew exactly what she was doing. But I thought to myself how sick and frail some asthmatics are when they really get debilitated. A smoke-filled room or puffing off of a cigarette could be ludicrous for someone like that. I thought about all the asthmatic kids that have to be so careful, and their parental watchdogs. I also said to myself, I hope Sara quits playing around and just stays away from smoke as much as possible.

"Listen, Henry, it's good to see ya, let's go sit down and have a bite to eat and talk for a while. I hate to do it, but we better talk some business, too. Have you been informed about anything yet, what's going on inside this nurse's body?"

"No, I just got in today. I was supposed to talk to the Major who spoke tonight, but you can bring me up to date on the inside story. I'll go and see him tomorrow," I smiled.

"Sure. Yeah, I have to talk to you. I'm glad you're going to be here with us. We can use your strategic mind and your experience."

"Sounds like war again, am I right?" I asked, almost afraid of the affirmative.

"Well, that's the possibility," George sighed.

"You mean likelihood," I replied.

"Come on, follow me, let's go get a bite to eat and then some rest. Hey, I'll bet I have some news that you're unaware of, that'll just knock you off your feet," George chuckled.

"What?" I raised my eyebrows.

"Females, that's what, they've infiltrated, say we have about two hundred in this district alone and thousands throughout."

But I told George I had him on this one. I had been working too, not sitting idle in some retirement camp, and I let him know I enjoyed women, their company and their intelligence. We grabbed some food and took it back to his headquarters. He wanted to talk about the serious stuff, what might occur and how we had to prepare, but I made him take a detour. So we just sat there and talked mostly about our success cases from the past.

CHAPTER 9

"The first thing we do Ellie, to treat your sinusitis, is open the passages that drain the sinus areas," said Dr. Wicker.

"How do you do that? Does it hurt?" asked Ellie, a soft-spoken, shy ten year old brunette with spiral curls like Shirley Temple.

"No, it can usually be done with decongestant medications and by breathing steam from a vaporizer. Then if that doesn't make it completely better, we have other methods that we can try. And drinking lots of water, can you do that Ellie?" coaxed the doctor.

"Uh huh. But what are sinuses and how do they get plugged up Doctor?" Ellie asked in a nasal tone as she twirled the ends of her hair with her fingers.

The doctor explained that she had something called an eth-moid sinus problem. Think of a sinus as a little cave or opening and eth-moid is just a name for one specific area. "It's about right here." Dr. Wicker pointed as she touched Ellie near the nose. "And if it gets congested or filled up with a bunch of stuff, you know, that stuff you have to keep blowing your nose to get rid of, well, then it can cause pain between the eyes, make your eyelids swell, like they are."

The doctor glanced toward Ellie's mother who sat next to her daughter. "And we think Mrs. Gibner, that in Ellie's case, as you suspected, the sinus condition may require getting her allergies under better control. So we have a lot of work to do. But Ellie, we know what to do to start making you feel better, okay." She touched her softly on the right shoulder. At that moment a nurse standing near the door explained that there was a phone call for the doctor.

Dr. Wicker stood up, "All right, we were just about through here." The doctor asked the nurse to explain where the pharmacy was located and how the outpatient clinic worked in relation to allergy testing and management, and to schedule another appointment in a week for Ellie. "Then I'll see you two in a week. Mrs. Gibner, if she doesn't begin to improve in a few days, or if you have any questions, just call."

Mrs. Gibner quickly thanked Dr. Wicker. He reminded her to push the liquids, "unsweetened preferably." Then he turned back and said, "Ellie, we're on the right track now, the medicine should help you feel better."

"Okay, bye."

While Clara, the nurse, explained a few things and answered some questions for Mrs. Gibner, a hospital aide in a blue, lengthy jacket walked by trying to find the clinic coordinator. "Excuse me," he said, "I'm from supplies and this is supposed to go to one of the pediatric nurses, is that you?" Clara accepted the box of respiratory supplies and said thank you.

When she finished up with Mrs. Gibner and Ellie, Clara walked down to the work-up room to see the next patient. Tammy managed the phones and the time schedule board, while Clara picked up a chart from the basket, looked at the name in the right hand corner and struggled to pronounce it. "Mister Dru-, Druserenski," Clara said as she looked at two men in business suits, and a woman and her two kids, who sat in chairs waiting to hear their names, along with several other asthmatics. One man stood up.

"Dru-ser-enski, how do you like that for a name?" He laughed.

"Oh it sounds all right. It's different." Clara smiled as the man walked toward her. "Would you follow me please?" gestured Clara.

"Certainly," he replied co-operatively.

"Just have a seat and take off your shoes please, so we can get your weight." He leaned down to untie his shoes. Clara glanced through the chart quickly to find the page that she needed and then asked, "Is this your first time here, Mr. Druserenski?"

"Just call me Glen. Yes it is. My doctor recommended this clinic and some of the education classes."

"Well good." She paused while she searched the room for her stethoscope. "Since this is your first time here, what we do in this room is weigh you, take your pulse and blood pressure and have you take a spirometry test. Now, I'll show you how to do that. It gives us an idea of what your breathing capacity is. Then, I'll see if the doctor is ready to see you."

"Oh, okay," he said.

"And you're here to see doctor who?" Clara asked.

"Dr. Loy," the patient answered. Clara checked to see what room number Dr. Loy occupied and wrote it in the lower left hand corner, along with the date, time, her initials and made a check mark by outpatient and spirometry test. "Now I need your age."

"Forty-eight," he replied matter-of-factly.

"And have you used an inhaler recently?"

"Yes, let's see, oh, about 11:00, no 11:30 this morning, I remember, just before I ate something." He patted his pudgy stomach.

Clara logged in the time, then said, "Step right up here."

Mr. Druserenski stepped up on the scale.

"It looks like 88.6 kilograms which is," she looked up at the conversion chart on the wall, "195 pounds."

The patient seemed puzzled at the reality of gaining a few pounds. The nurse told him to have a seat and put his shoes back on. Then she reached out and took a hold of his right hand. "Let me get your pulse." She placed her index and middle finger over his radial pulse and listened while looking at the second hand on her watch. After fifteen seconds passed, she jotted down seventy-six.

Next, Clara maneuvered a blood pressure cuff around Mr. Druserenski's right, upper arm. With her stethoscope in place, she pumped the black rubber bulb, then released it slowly until she heard a thump. She made a mental note of the systolic number.   When she no longer heard the pulsating sound, she deflated the cuff, unraveled it, put the stethoscope back around her neck and then wrote down the two numbers.

"That's 124 over 76," Clara said. "Looks fine, not a high blood pressure at all."

"Well, that's about right for me."   He sounded reassured.

"Is it?" Clara asked as she folded the cuff.

"Yes, I usually run about 126 or 130."

"Now I need you to do one more thing. Have you ever taken the spirometer test before?" Clara asked.

"Yes I know how to do it, but this one looks a little different than the one they used at St. Peter's Hospital. I just take a deep breath, right, and blow?" He inhaled and exhaled.

"That's right. You want to take a real deep breath, blow as hard and as long as you can. Here, you hold this, wait and let me put this on your nose and this in here. All right, we're all set."

Mr. Druserenski breathed deeply, pursed his lips over the circular shaped mouth piece and blew into it. Afterward he coughed and remarked in a weak voice, almost a whisper, "That hurts, you know."

"Does it?   You mean your lungs as you breathed deeply?" Clara placed her hand on his chest.

"Yeah, there's a pain," he squinted.

"A pain, where exactly?" Clara tried to pinpoint the location and type of pain, but the patient explained that it hurt all throughout his lungs as he exhaled.

"Well, we'll let the doctor know that." Clara patted Mr. Druserenski on the back gently. "That's why you're here, to find out what's wrong and how we can help."

"Okay," he sighed and sat down, with a sad expression on his face. After Clara finished writing down a few things, she tried to reassure him, then excused herself. She returned a minute later.

"All right, just follow me right down here to room number three. Have a seat and Dr. Loy will be right in." Mr. Druserenski followed her and walked into the room.

"Thank you Nurse."

"Well, I hope you start feeling better. Take care,"

Clara said as she walked back toward the sitting room to work up the next patient.

Max, a fourteen year old boy had been in gym class when an asthma attack occurred. Although he appeared to be only wheezing mildly at this time, it was obvious that he had just suffered an attack. He appeared upset and tired and sat with his fists on the chair so that he could brace himself as he leaned forward to get more comfortable. His mother looked extremely concerned. Clara escorted the two of them to the treatment room.

Two hours later, Clara looked at her watch, stepped around the corner to find out if any charts or people sat in the waiting room. She walked back, straightened up the two chairs and picked up a Kleenex off the floor and tossed it into the wastebasket. She took her calculator and put it in her pocket, then headed for the receptionist's desk.

"See you Monday Andrea. Jo Alice, say bye to Maria."

"See you later Clara." Andrea waved.

"Bye, have a nice weekend." Jo Alice reached for the telephone and waved goodbye while Clara smiled back.

Then Clara sneezed and as she walked away, she heard her friends simultaneously say, "Gesundheit." She recalled a German friend from her childhood who had informed her that the word actually is used to wish a person good health, not say "bless you," as she had assumed.

CHAPTER 10

"Henry," George nagged. "We have to discuss this, we're running out of time and a lot of the other reactors want to know if you're with us or not. Remember, pals, buddies, like we used to say. I can't figure out what's going on in that mind of yours, you agreed that you wouldn't sit by passively while the enemy attacked. Right?" prodded George.

"That's what I said, I suppose, but there's more to it than that, George, and I'm not sure I can make you or the rest of them understand."

"Understand what? For Pete's sake, if you tell me, I can let you know if I understand or not."

"George, it's not a simple matter. If I just had a little more time, maybe I could think of a way," I hedged.

But George got serious all of a sudden and emphasized that time kept ticking by and told me that I would have to tell him what was bothering me so that I could clear the air once and for all. "Tomorrow, Henry, that's it," he said to me. "I got word that all of the high risk factors will be in full swing. They're going to need us Henry."

"Okay George, I'll be there, but remember what you said about believing in my strategic mind and especially my experience. I want to plant that idea firmly in your head, because there may come a time when I need you to rely on a certain way do things, even if it goes beyond orders from some high-ranking superiors. Now I need to know if you're with me!" I looked dead into my friend's eyes.

"Well, can't say that I understand completely, but I'm registering what you tell me. I'm taking it to heart, Henry, okay pal? Will that do for now? Unless you want to elaborate," he coaxed.

"I think we've said enough for now. Let's go locate those two sources you have and do some digging and see if we can get any more information, what do you say?" I asked.

"All right. Let's go."

"This way, we'll go check with the Vessel Patrol Force," directed George.

As we moved about in Clara's circulation, we discussed the old days and how much progress had been made in the area of understanding immunology and ways to prevent diseases.

"The plague, polio, typhoid fever, measles, mumps, rabies, infectious pathogens, those all used to be the main problems," I pointed out.

"Yeah, nowadays, it's all sorts of different antigens, still have some deadly viruses, bacterial battles, self-destructive lifestyles, and the AIDS epidemic that we have to fight. I've been hearing some strange things lately, as if we're regressing occasionally due to shortages of vaccines, and those unexpected over-reactive cases. There was a young boy in Georgia who became an invalid after his shots. It caused a panic, and before you knew it, the whole community, some people all over the world, after the press got wind of it, didn't have any faith anymore in the immunization process. I don't know what the solution is there do you?" asked George.

"It's a tough one George, I don't know. It's a real dilemma. I've done some research on that though. Seems like we just have to protect against epidemics and yet for the one in a million or one in 300,000 that gets stuck with death or a permanent disability, it doesn't seem fair, the worst kind of tragedy happens," I rationalized.

"Say, did you ever wish you were human?" He asked me another question.

"What, and have to learn to adapt to that crazy world out there, no thanks. Those humans can be complicated creatures sometimes. Besides, I couldn't get used to the multi-shaded or shaven hairstyles or some of the ridiculous crime rates. I'll stay put, right here inside my little human biological environment. At least in here I know what I'm up against. That world scares me sometimes, but I think it shows so much promise, you know, the American dream and all that. I've seen it happen," I elaborated, "and the people out there, well you know how terrific and good-hearted some of them can be. I guess it's the old concept of good versus evil that frightens or baffles me more than anything," I rambled on.

Then George started to clue me in on what he heard a professor at Yale say once at a lecture, and it made a lot of sense. It dealt with the subject of fear.

The professor emphasized the profound notion that people are never really free of the fear of something unless the individual is also free of the fear associated with it. In other words, he meant to say, that the perception of a threat can be just as harmful as the real threat.

I thought about Sara's adaptation to smoke and her victory over the fear and threat of what smoke might do to her as far as causing an asthma attack, and the way she managed to utilize relaxation techniques sometimes to avoid panicking during her worst attacks.

"Hmm," I scratched my head. "I think Dr. Hansel's work was profound, yet simplistic, in a way. After all, adapting is supposed to be a basic phenomenon of humans as well as animals. Yeah, I've read all about Dr. Hansel's and Dr. Brownie's theories and research on stress and adaptation. Did you ever get to hear them speak?" I asked.

"Yes, I did see Dr. Hansel once, a year before he passed away, and believe me, it was fascinating. Went with a medical technologist to a seminar convention one day. She was scurrying around looking for answers, fluctuating between more traditional treatment and the more extreme ecologically based emphasis. God Henry, what a day. You never would have believed it if you hadn't seen it with your own eyes. All day Saturday, we sat through speaker after speaker, at this spectacular hotel in Reno. You're aware of the difference, right, between more conservative allergists and what they call clinical ecologists? And then the psychologists, some who lean toward physiological maladaptations, others who lean toward psychological origins in regards to disease states?"

"Yes George, what happened?" I asked excitedly. I listened in awe while my buddy talked about history being made that day. A big debate had taken place.

"Dr. Hansel was there, more as a mediator than anything else. Both sides had provided lectures and presented patients who had been treated by all different types of therapies. Some of them told the saddest stories. People who even moved out of their houses and searched for, or constructed, a less allergenic environment. And the angry ones, people who had been told over and over again, that it was all in their head, that their allergies or intolerances, their multitude of physiological responses didn't even exist. (That we, antibodies, didn't even exist or do our jobs.) Henry, it was pathetic at times."

I told him to continue.

"Anyway, philosophical mediators and Dr. Hansel were working throughout the day, and by dusk they had managed to bring about what seemed to be the impossible. Everyone, I mean everyone, was shaking hands. I don't know how they did it. All of the leftist psychologists shaking hands with the right-winged ones. Can you imagine, Freudians and Jungian types merging? Immunologists shared information and kept an open ear to all of the various theories. Clinical psychologists and other allergists met in one room and debated hot issues. Everyone listened to the other side of the story, and agreed to merge forces, for the sake of the patients. Afterwards, there was an inspiring celebration. You should have seen their faces, the happiness, the peace, and relief. I felt as if I was watching a post-war celebration. What a day!" George took a deep breath; then sighed.

At this point, I felt utterly bewildered by George's long, highly fabricated speech. I did, however, let him finish before saying something about the way he always managed to throw in his own happy ending tales, because I truly liked George's "stories."

"Yeah, even the allergic victims themselves, they promised to concentrate on all areas of health education: good sound nutrition, adequate rest and relaxation, meds, exercise, sexuality, emotional issues, and certain do's and don'ts that allergic individuals have to pay attention to. Also, adequate interests, purpose in life and social support."

"Social support?" I wanted him to elaborate.

"A medical sociologist said that boredom and loneliness can be contributing factors in a person's illness or ability to improve. He reminded us how a lot of allergic/asthmatic kids can't have pet companions like other kids. That all makes a difference."

Everyone at the convention agreed on and emphasized the connection between the body and mind, and the remarkable potential which people have to help themselves toward an optimum point with conscientious, persistent rehabilitative effort and support. The allergic and asthmatic individuals vowed to work on internal control as well as external circumstances." He rambled on enthusiastically. "They explained that realistic limitations may make it more difficult for some people, but they acknowledged the fact that there was always an optimal level of functioning to strive for."

"Say, George, uh buddy." He still looked like he was daydreaming, actually reliving the event. (I thought to myself, you sure can be a real Danny Kaye-Walter Mitty character sometimes.) "You know, I sure don't recall hearing anything about this historical, monumental convention, and being an antibody you'd think I'd know if something like this took place. Are you certain about this unforgettable day in history, that it took place exactly like you said?" I added a patronizing tone of voice, without meaning to.

George frowned and turned toward me with a shameful look on his face. "Ah Henry, I'm sorry. I got a little carried away again, didn't I? Well darn it, it doesn't hurt to dream, does it? I think we're all getting closer to answers and working together, it might happen someday. I'm sorry bud, for giving you all that fairy tale stuff. Why didn't you stop me, let me carry on that way, like an old fool? But the convention Henry, it happened, just not quite like I told it."

I empathized with him. "I know George, we all want to hope for the best. And they are getting to the bottom of things with better research and more understanding health care. Things will work out. It just takes a while."

"I don't know," he said sadly, "sometimes I just wonder about it all, about my life, my job, you know? Last month I had to work on this transplant case, was lucky to escape with my old life. Well, you know how tricky it is with those transplant cases, you've endured some."

"Yeah, a few. I know how dangerous they are. You've had one recently huh? Did the person make it?" I asked, hoping the victim lived.

"Not this one, I'm afraid. I don't even know what I was doing there, since I'm an allergy specialist, but they transferred me anyway. Was a darn shame too. We fought like crazy for that little guy. Sometimes, I just...," he began to cry, but held back, "I uh, just wouldn't work another one of those, that's all I know. I'd quit first."

"Yeah, I know George, me too. How old?"

"Only six." George described the loss, how a bunch of phagos, macros and lymphos worked with the antibody troops. But the little boy, Berry, died anyway. Later, some high-rankers that weren't even at the death scene, but had given the orders then escaped, were to be court-martialed. The charges were poor judgment. They pleaded 'rejection phenomenon' and got off. But there were a lot of education classes after that, all concerning overreaction, personal liability, and how nobody can ever escape it. All of the transplant specialists had to take the classes. Recommended them for everyone else too."

"I heard about this George, except that you were involved. I didn't know you were there. It must have been a close call then, hmm?"

"Believe me, it was. There were only a few of us that reached the conclusion in time, that we had to retreat or die, that's what it came down to Henry. We couldn't persuade the others, so we waited for a blood transfusion one day and got out by passive transfer. Henry, it just wasn't my time to go yet. I felt like a real coward that day. But I wish it could have been different. I wish it with all my heart. In a sense, I guess, I felt somewhat of a rebel too, knowing the truth of the matter, not willing to follow the old train of thought."

"There weren't any survivors left, were there?" I asked.

"No, not the ones who stayed. It was one of those cases that meant victory or all out defeat for everyone. We all lost that day. A sad day in history."

I thought to myself, maybe it's not going to be so hard to make George understand after all. My friend was feeling a great deal of pain, but I didn't really know what to say, so I didn't say anything. After that conversation though, I felt relieved and more comfortable around him. Some of the anxiety had disappeared.

"Here he is, Vessel Patrol Officer Geno Getson. Geno, how's it going, busy tonight?" George switched moods and smiled.

"A little more than usual, not too bad, George, what are you up to?" The patrolbody tipped his hat.

"I need to find Privates Richey and Porter, you know where they are? This is a friend of mine, Sergeant Henry Halt, he's new on this case." He introduced us.

"Hi. Pleasure." He saluted me.

"Hi." I smiled and offered my hand.

"Well, Richey's out on pollen grain watch and Porter's on dog dander duty. Always a little action there." Geno stuck his hands in his pockets.

"What time are they reporting in?"

"At 2200 hours," Geno said.

"Okay, listen, will you tell them George wants to talk to them, to stop by the cell tonight, nothing important. Just want to ask them something."

"Sure will. Are you sure you don't want me to leave a message of any sort?" Geno coaxed.

"No, I just want to ask them about switching one day next week with Henry and myself. Thanks. See you later," said George.

"Hey George, do you think he'd know anything?"

"I wouldn't want to ask him. They say he reports everything. I mean everything and anything out of the ordinary. I don't trust the guy. He's too much like a robot. Think he's trying to brown-nose his way up to Head Patrol Officer, but any way he can."

"Hmm. Great." I answered sarcastically.

At 10:30 p.m. sharp, there was a knock at George's membrane. He found out what he wanted to know, but couldn't figure out what the exact danger was yet. Clara planned to go camping over the weekend with her husband. They mentioned horseback riding in a conversation last week. That's the only thing George could think of. She talked about reactions before, but says she's got plenty of meds. Richey and Porter were to keep their ears open. He said goodnight and then we all decided to get some rest.

"We'll talk to Major Borline tomorrow. He lives right next door. He's a good one to talk to," George explained as I stood at his cell door.

"Okay George, you know the situation around here better than I do."

We both retired. My eyes were closed, but I kept trying to piece things together, figure out if we were missing something, what the true dangers might be. I thought about George's ordeal and comments that he had made today. I knew we were on the same wavelength now, whereas, before, I wasn't certain. I fell asleep within the half hour. I was exhausted.

CHAPTER 11

Early in the morning, the Major heard us knocking at his membrane. "Sergeant George, I'm glad you're here. I've got to clue you in on some things." Major Borline welcomed us.

"How much time is left before we know what the source of the problem is?" asked George.

"Well, we won't know until it hits her, but we've narrowed down the possibilities. Who's your friend, Sergeant George?" The Major had started addressing George by using his first name as his last long ago, and never stopped, for some reason.

"Oh, this is Sergeant Henry Halt. Henry, Major Borline. He's with us all the way, Sir." George glanced at me with a piercing look.

"Hello, Major Borline, nice to meet you." I smiled and offered my hand.

"So, Sergeant Henry, you're going to give us some extra help? Well, we're probably going to need you. Glad you're here. Now let's sit down. Like I was saying, the foreigners we'll be looking for are: pollen, mold, etc. She's been overdosing on some of her favorite foods too, so watch that. The digestive reactors have battled it out the last day or so due to a large milk shake. I've got Sergeant Deb Doss and her specialty troop tracking food allergy threats, since so many well-intended, but misguided operatives, are always setting off false alarms and causing havoc.

The monthly hormonal shifts are causing the reactors to behave hyper-sensitively, too. Also, keep an eye out for insect, bee or snake bites. That's a possibility since she's planning a hike in the foothills. It's rare, but it could happen. Other than that, perhaps the exercise-induced problem, but that's usually controlled by her inhalers."

The Major then explained that he would spend the next couple of hours preparing the regiments, assigning posts and informing the troops about the anticipation of a severe reaction. He made it clear, without prompting from either George or myself, that no fighting or explosive reactions were appropriate unless he gave the orders.

He said very seriously to us, "Remember, this is a Code Red Emergency Alert. They've got to be ready. Expect orders from Sergeant Birlly, myself, or other commanders on duty. Oh, the rest of the IgE battalion, they'll have orders to get ready to lock onto their specific antigens. Captain Kale will be there to give the explosive orders. Sergeant George, make sure we have a stocked supply of histamine-packed granules ready. She's leaving about 0900 hours. That gives us at least three hours to have everyone man their battle stations. Of course the B and T Cell regiments are on alert too and all of the Granulocyte regiments are geared up. It's up to us to protect her." He looked dead at us. "Sergeant Henry, George, may God be with us."

"Yes Sir," George said. I saluted and said the same. "We're on our way Sir."

I paused on my way out, wanted to ask the Major something, but felt a nudge from George and changed my mind.

"We'll be ready for whatever it is. We all want to save her, right Sir?" George risked prolonging our stay and emphasizing the issue I wanted to stress, saving the girl rather than destroying her.

"Absolutely," agreed the Major. Now, I'm headed over to the T and B regiments, I've got to make absolutely certain that they're standing by. I'll get back to you later; let's say ten-hundred hours."

George grabbed my arm and we hurriedly began to organize Clara's self-defense troops.

CHAPTER 12

"What a beautiful morning. It's just perfect. Bret, wake up." Clara nudged her husband, but he failed to respond, except to twitch his right foot.

Clara stepped out of bed, opened the front door, glanced at the sky and took a few deep breaths. The cool morning air filled her nostrils. She noticed the clear sky, the quietness, and watched the sparrows bathing in the birdbath while some of them scrounged around on the ground for food particles. While bending over to pick up the newspaper, she read the headlines.

"SURGEON COMES FORWARD AFTER TWENTY-NINE YEARS. HIS BOOK, *JFK: A CONSPIRACY OF SILENCE*, REVEALS ASTOUNDING FACTS."

After turning off the porch light, she walked to the kitchen and tossed the paper on the table. "Honey," she walked into the bedroom. "Time to get up. Remember, you said we'd leave by nine or so."

Bret groaned and turned over on his right side.

"I'll fix up some scrambled eggs and toast. You have to wake up, or it'll be the cold wash rag treatment," she threatened.

He opened his eyes widely. "I think it's about time we got going, don't you sweetheart? I'll go jump in the shower. Do you think I need to shave?"

Clara laughed at his abrupt alertness. "It's amazing how you wake up so fast sometimes. Shave? Let me feel your whiskers." She sat on the side of the bed, placed her right hand on his cheek and rubbed her palm against his face. He put his arms around her and kissed her. Clara nestled back down next to him. They embraced and began to childishly wrestle with each other.

"Bret! Bret! Stop, you're tickling me." Clara tried to make him stop.

"Hmm?" He kissed her neck, just below the left earlobe.

"Don't shave. I like your whiskers."

"And I like you. In fact, I love you."

"Oh I love you so much. I can never say it enough." After breakfast, Clara tried, discreetly, to hurry Bret along, so they could leave for the anticipated weekend adventure.

"Hey, by the way," Clara said, "You're supposed to cuddle with me under the stars tonight, not today in an ordinary bed. Remember? A bottle of lemonade and the 'sky as our ceiling'."

"Who said I forgot? I'll get the lemonade out of the refrigerator right now." He walked toward the kitchen. "I'll get the cheese spread and crackers now too." He yelled, "Are you ready for a good long hike, honey?"

"Yeah, I'm ready. Do you think we'll see any deer? Roy and Val," she shouted, "were up there a couple of weeks ago, not that park, but one close by and they saw some Mule deer. I asked them to go, but Val had a wedding to go to. Besides, it will be fun with just us."

As he finished up packing a few more items from the kitchen he headed for the bedroom. "I don't know, we could see some deer," he answered. "Did you decide yet on the horseback riding or not?"

"I think I want to go Bret, if you do. I'll take my medicine along, and if I sneeze, I'll just sneeze it out. I've got plenty of tissues and antihistamines, and my inhalers of course. Oh, and the anaphylactic kit, it's in the first aid pack."

Clara fed her dog Harvey. Julian, a friend, agreed to look after him for the weekend. One last stroke of love by his masters and Bret and Clara were in the jeep driving toward Golden. Clara searched the map in her hand for

Pine exit. Once they found it, they could follow that road into Roundup State Park.

"Hey, it says here that the park 'is noted for a wide variety of wildlife, including deer, bear, mountain lion and wild turkey.' I'd love to see a lion." She continued to read. "Hiking/equestrian trails have been located on the perimeter of major wildlife habitat areas so as to allow the public to view the animals in their natural setting, yet not to disturb them. Therefore, it is of prime importance for the park user to stay on the trails that are provided. The park user should also be aware..." She stopped suddenly and read silently, then blurted out, "Listen to this, 'the park user should also be aware that the Diamond Back rattlesnake is found throughout the park, so caution should be exercised during the warm season'."

"You saw one before up here, didn't you?"

"Yeah, remember, I told you about it. I heard it. It was off the trail directly to the left of where I stepped. I looked and didn't see anything, but we ran out of there. You should have seen how scared Ron was. Remember, that day I went with Ron and June last year?"

"I remember. But you didn't see any more after that or hear any?"

"No, that was it."

"What did the rattle sound like?"

"Just like a rattle. Like someone shaking a baby's rattle, maybe a little faster than usual," she explained.

"Hmm. There it is, Pine Road."

"I see it. It's a perfect day, too. Let me get the suntan lotion. It's warm already." She reached in the glove compartment and found a small tube of Coppertone and her make-up bag with her medicine inside. "Is the first aid kit still in the trunk?"

Bret decided to park under a shady tree. Clara grabbed items from the back seat as he unloaded the trunk. He scattered everything on the ground. Off to the left, the first aid kit caught his eye. He told Clara to stick it in her backpack.

"It's great having my very own EMT around. This kit has everything. You really stuffed it." After some organizing, and changing into hiking shoes, the two of them began to hike along the sloped dirt trail. Bret held a map in his hand that designated which direction to follow in order to find the camping area. The bright sun and dry air was refreshing. Clara thought to herself, finally, we're here. "God I love the outdoors. It's so beautiful and peaceful." Bret shared his wife's exact thoughts.

CHAPTER 13

"It's windy today, huh. I hate windy days," Clara said.
"Why?"

"I don't know, unless I'm flying a kite, I just never liked the wind. I can't seem to think straight in it, and it makes my ears hurt." She stopped and let the backpack slide down off of her shoulders. "Here, wait sweetie, I'm going to put some Kleenex in them, let's stop for just a second."

"Nag, nag, nag." Bret said facetiously.

Clara, on the other hand, took his comments seriously. "I'm not nagging, just telling you something, there's a difference." After tearing off a small piece of tissue, she formed two little round balls and inserted them in each ear. "There, that's better."

"All set?" He hoisted her blue backpack up over her shoulders.

"Know what?" Clara said.

"What?"

"I keep thinking about the movie last night. The last part was pretty tough to digest, wasn't it?"

"What do you mean?"

"Well, it was such a parallel. There's her boyfriend, so happy, calling to tell her that they finally got Carnegie Hall, the first time for a jazz singer, a dream come true. And there she is, hugging the dead and bloody piano man. All because she had to go and get messed up again. It was so tragic."

"Yeah, I wonder what happened next, but I guess we'll never know, since a certain person had to get up and turn the TV off." He tried to swat a fly that had landed on his left arm.

"Well, I'm sorry, but I just couldn't watch it anymore. They always do that. It couldn't end happily. She should have made it. (What's with all these flying, hopping grasshoppers? She mumbled to herself.) I know that they had to depict reality. Drug addiction is a tough thing to beat and I guess Billie Holiday was just one of the unlucky ones. It's a shame, so many lives are ruined, so many broken dreams, just because some people have to abuse drugs and alcohol."

"Well, you know better than anyone else, Clara, with your mom."

"I know. It hurts so bad sometimes. I wish she could have a different kind of life, a healthy life. She's so beautiful in so many ways. And yet, we have to watch her head down a dead-end street." They hiked along the trail, silent for a few minutes.

"Here, let's go to the right here." Bret pointed.

"Okay, you're the leader."

They both made an angular turn and continued hiking up a trail called Wild Arrow. "But you know what, I think I understand alcoholism a lot better these days. How it just ruined aspects of my mom's life." Her words sounded choppy. She took a deep breath and huffed and puffed while climbing as the slope steepened.

"Well, you know you don't have to tell me, the AA veteran."

Clara smiled and took another deep breath. "You know, if you think about it, some of the nicest people around, the most sensitive, creative, famous, or even prominent people in the world are alcoholics or past alcoholics. Like Mom and Dad, I feel for them. But I sure do feel for innocent victims, too, because of some of those neat, but dangerous people. The thing I always worried most about was my parents' drinking and driving. Why is it that when someone is hurting or heading toward self-destruction, they refuse to get help and work toward getting better? I want her to get well, to stop drinking so much and stop smoking herself to death. Can I sit down just for a second, okay?" Feeling exhausted, Clara noticed a large rock and headed for it.

Bret teased, "Can't talk and walk at the same time, you know what they say."

"I know, I know. I wish I had the money. I'd send her to one of those fancy health resorts or well-known rehabilitation centers, or I guess if she'd just go to AA. And now she's coughing so much with that evil smoking habit. Poor Mom, she's always sick. I always wished for some magic power so I could give her better health, a better life."

"I like your mom too, a lot, but I hate to see her like this." He shook his head from side to side.

Clara became pensive and visions of last month when her mom had adverse reactions to some drugs haunted her. She had found her mom sleepy and sick, mumbling about taking some pills. Scared, but not panicky, Clara dialed 911 and the dispatcher told her he would send an ambulance right away. Clara realized later, that her mom would have died if she had not found her in time.

Attempting to sound positive, Clara said, "But Mom's been trying to cut down on her drinking. I just spoke to her the other day and she's eating a little better, orders by her doctor."

"Good. Hey, how come your dad can handle his drinking without getting sick?"

"I don't know. He just does. I think it's because he eats better than mom and gets some nutrition, mostly home cooking, whereas mom seems to eat just sandwiches and supper once and awhile. And I think, you know, the male versus female biology, hormones, and way of life, Mom worries about everything and dad just says 'such is life' and takes things in stride."

"Hmm. That sounds like your dad."

"Now, let's talk about our hiking trip!" Clara said excitedly.

"I'm all for that."

"We're going to hike up to the camping area, right?"

"Right!" Bret affirmed.

"Then get set up for the night, right?"

"Right!"

"Then go over to the stables right, and ride a horse."

"We'll try anyway, it's been a while you know, and if you're sure you won't get sick on me."

"Then what?" asked Clara.

"I don't know," he paused. "Maybe walk some more, or get out the grill and cook supper, or the Scrabble game or cards and see if you can beat me. And then get ready for our bottle of lemonade and night under the stars."

"Sounds romantic to me. Will you really play Scrabble? Usually, I have to beg you."

"Yeah, if we're not too tired from everything else, sure."

"Okay. All it takes is a little mind power anyway and enough energy to pick up the letters." Clara's wheezing got louder.

"You sound like you're having troubles."

"Yeah, I need to spray. I can't walk and talk at the same time, and this altitude isn't helping." Clara reached into her pockets for her inhaler device and tiny bottle of eye drops. After shaking the inhaler and exhaling, simultaneously, she put her lips around the opening and inhaled as she pressed down. She soon took a second puff.

After a brief rest, they hiked past a sign posted on a fence to their right which read: "RIFLE RANGE: KEEP OUT." Downtown Denver and three small manmade lakes were clearly visible as they reached the peak of a vista point.

After passing another sign which pointed toward GABLE'S STABLES, Clara stepped quickly to the left to avoid a pile of dried up horse manure. The dirt trail became sandy, then rocky again, and zigzagged in a north and south direction, mostly sloping upward, but occasionally easing with a brief downhill slope. A quiet mood fell upon Clara and Bret as the wind made the pine trees sway. The only sounds were a few buzzing bees, and several birds chirping in the distance. They hiked another three-fourths of a mile and had to decide which trail to take.

"According to this, we can take Hayride, the long way around, or turn right toward the campsite with Indianhead. What do you think, walk straight to it, save time so we can go horseback riding?"

"Sure," agreed Bret, "that sounds good."

It was only another half a mile until they reached the campsite. The temperature exceeded ninety degrees, and the perspiration dropped off of their faces as they hiked and stopped occasionally to sip cold water from a yellow picnic jug. Suddenly, Bret stopped and pointed, trying to get Clara's attention, but she kept looking down at her feet while walking until she finally glanced up and saw him standing perfectly still.

"There. Look," he whispered and stared at a large gray deer very close by. The deer stood motionless and stared back.

"Oh, how gorgeous. He's so neat." Clara whispered. "Look at him look right at us, like wanting to ask us what the heck we're doing here."

"Well, this is his territory." They both admired the wild animal for a few more moments, then hiked until they reached a sign with an arrow on it, designating that the campsite veered directly to the left. A green water pump off to the right also caught their attention.

"Look, we have extra water! Let's go try it." Excitedly they neared the water pump, but then both of them were startled by a hornet that kept whizzing by. Clara screamed the first time it flew by her.

"Clara, don't scream! It will just attract its attention."

"I know. But it scared me." She began to walk backward away from the pump. "You get the water. I'm going to check out the campsite. Be careful." She ran toward a grassy area and yelled, "Bye."

Bret proceeded calmly, but cautiously, ignoring the bee. He placed both hands on the long slender handle and pushed it downward and pulled it back up again, until the water gushed out from the green pump. After dropping his backpack to the ground, he searched for a small pink picnic jug. He filled the jug to the top, tasted the water, which was quite cold. Then he walked over to the campsite where Clara had already made herself at home.

"Did you have any bee problems?"

"Nope. No problems. I think the little rascal is gone." He set his backpack down. "Hey, this is nice here, huh?"

"It's beautiful, all this open space, I love it."

He noticed the beauty and solitude of the location. They were surrounded by a few trees, and grassy open areas to the east and north of them. Several pieces of driftwood had been skillfully placed around a grill.

"They even have a grill ready for us, and some driftwood to sit on. This is perfect. Looks like someone was here just recently."

"Sure does, doesn't it? Maybe yesterday." He walked over to Clara and sat next to her. He hugged her and she wrapped her arms around him. They kissed several times. Then he asked, "Are you going to help me set up the tent?"

"Sure." But neither one of them moved. After another long kiss, Bret smiled and began to stare into Clara's ocean-blue eyes.

"You know what?"

"What?" Clara wondered if something romantic was coming.

"I could remain lost forever in these mountains with you."

"Me too. God I love you." She kissed him passionately again. "No wait. The idea would be, to be found forever, and together, not lost," Clara said seriously.

He laughed, "Okay, okay. Found then, and together. Let's get this tent set up."

CHAPTER 14

"Major! Major!" We heard Corporeal Geno Getson yell as he pounded on Major Borline's membrane. He responded immediately. Corporeal Getson explained, "I've sounded the alarms. Sir, this could be it, foreigners have been spotted in the bloodstream! She's on a horse right now!"

"Foolish woman. I knew she'd have trouble with that horse idea. What the heck's she waiting for? Why doesn't she take her medicine? Give orders to react, but only accordingly, with reasonable due progression. Any doubts or concerns, get back to me first. Corporeal Getson, tell Sergeants Henry and George to get up to those nasal and bronchial tube lines, to help wherever they can. And Corporeal Getson, keep watch for Code Red Emergency Status. We're going to prevent or combat against any critical ordeals here. I like this little lady, understand?" His voice was gruff and commanding.

"Yes Sir! Got it Sir!" He saluted. Next, we heard someone pounding on our membrane. We all saluted each other and prepared ourselves mentally for battle.

Here's a little secret I'll share with you. The weakness in our immune army stems from the fact that we're always playing defense in these wars, never making the first preventive move. We can't, because we're reactors, counter attackers. Once the barrier is broken and the plasma cells fire the signal, that's when we act and then we overdue it.

George and I circulated up to the swollen bronchial tubes as ordered. We overheard the sinister intruders. The creeps were boasting about how they infiltrated. Most of them sifted through the nasal membranes, others by mouth. Keep in mind, this was just one location in the body; they were probably everywhere by now.

One little sneak, named Vance, started jabbing at one of Clara's cell membranes. "Hey: Vernie, Carlos, Tobie, Kristie, Kath, c'mon. Dig in! Let's set our attackers in action! Where's Ronnie and Karin? Let's go, this is what we're here for! The bosses aren't around. I'm not waitin' for any orders. They'd want us to tear into her anyway."

At that moment, George and I gritted our teeth and watched from a distance as our surface antibodies decided they had taken enough from the heartless enemies, and it was time to react.

"Neutralize!" One of our commanders ordered.

"Kill! Kill!" The antigen named Vernie yelled.

I found myself shouting back orders too, so we could counterattack and neutralize, as I lunged out at one of the antibodies. George was directly behind me cursing the relentless little creatures and charging too. We were holding our own when a skinny, mean antigen conked us on the head.

"Hon," Clara blinked her itching, red, swollen eyes and sniffled constantly as she spoke. "I've got to stop for a minute. Whoa, Wildfire, Whoa." The chocolate brown horse listened to her command, slowed down, and came to a halt. Bret turned his head, just for a second, but realized he was very close to a barbed wire fence to the right, so he looked straight ahead and guided the horse to the left, until he could stop. "What's the matter?" he shouted.

"What do you mean, what's the matter, the usual," Clara said sarcastically, but not loud enough for him to hear. "I'm having a sneezing, wheezing fit. Can't breathe and my eyes are killing me. I need water and my medicine." She spoke loudly now.

"Geez, look at your right eye, it's almost swollen shut Clara." Bret held onto his horse, dismounted, then walked back to Clara. "Here, hold onto these, I'll get the water out. Didn't you take something before we left? My God, you should see your eyes." He hurried to find the jug.

"Wait a second. I, I can't talk right now." She put the reigns in one hand and reached into her pocket for her inhaler. She went through the process, very quickly, of inhaling a dose of medication. She tried to attend to the horses. They were quiet but restless. However, she couldn't see very well, due to the condition of her eyes.

"Here." He handed her the water and grabbed the reins. "Now, what do you have to take, an antihistamine?"

"Yeah. And my eye drops. This makes me so mad!" She sipped some water and swallowed an antihistamine capsule. "Guess I messed up. I thought maybe I wouldn't have that much trouble if I wore gloves and used just the one preventive inhaler. Obviously, I was wrong. Maybe the inhaler was on zero doses already." She blew her nose several times on a tissue she had found.

Next, she proceeded to place two drops of liquid medicine into her eyes to reduce the itching and redness.

She apologized again. "Sorry about this. But you know what, at least it goes away about as fast as it comes on. I hope. That's what happened anyway, a couple of years ago when I went riding with Liz and her cousin Cheryl. I didn't even take anything that day. It just acted up; then subsided about an hour after I got off the horse."

"Yeah, well, it might settle down. But, apparently, today you needed that antihistamine," he said seriously. "You couldn't have some kind of curable illness, you have to have allergies."

"Well, excuse me. I didn't pick my health problem. I cannot help it if I have wild and crazy antibodies wandering around in my body," Clara responded.

"Are you ready to go now?"

"I'm ready."

"Did you hear that, Henry, she called us wild and crazy."

"Yeah, yeah, I heard. Oh my aching head. How long have we been out?" He rubbed the back of his head.

"I don't know for sure. Long enough, evidently. Everything's looking calmer again. Let's check out the damage and report back to the Major."

"Maybe that was it, Sergeant Henry, what do you think, the big scare?"

I had to laugh, George calling me Sergeant Henry. "Don't know Sergeant George, we'll have to wait and see."

"Yeah, we sure don't want to take any chances, be left off guard," his buddy agreed.

Bret helped position Clara's backpack and asked if she wanted to head back.

"No. I want to follow the trail around. I'll be all right. I'll probably get a little sleepy later with this pill though. Okay, let's go." She steadied herself on the horse as she nudged her shoes into the stirrups more securely.

"Sure, if you're ready. Can you see now?"

"Yes. My left eye's fine. The other one will get better soon."

"Well, be careful."

"I will. If I have to stop for something, I'll say so, but I should be all right now." She tried to reassure him.

"Hi-Ho Silver, and a way we go," he joked. Clara and Bret both laughed as they rode along. After the horseback ride, they hiked back to their campsite.

CHAPTER 15

"Let's just sit here for a little while. It's so peaceful." Clara straightened out her sleeping bag and laid it on the ground. "I knew I'd get sleepy with that pill I took. Gosh, I can't believe we did it, rode a horse. Can you?"

"Yeah I can believe it all right, even feel it. In fact, at this moment my rear-end is reminding me of the bumpy ride. Seems to me it didn't ache this much back when I was a kid and rode a horse." He snuggled up next to Clara and put his arm around her.

"Hey, do you think our lives are too fast-paced?" she asked, then added, "I mean, don't you ever wonder about living a different kind of life?"

"Well, sure I do. Sometimes I think about all of the different kinds of lives, occupations in the world. You know, upper class, us stuck in the middle class, people who live in poverty, maybe living somewhere else, maybe on a ranch, or running our own business or something like that. What about you, hon?"

After a few seconds of thought, Clara answered assuredly, "I'd be a musician, or writer, someone who never gives up on that inner voice, or motivation to follow that musical or creative unique quality about myself. Know what I mean?"

He took a sip of water from the jug then offered it to Clara. "I know what you mean, exactly." He mentioned how the creative ones usually live painful lives, though, kind of a roller-coaster existence, but figure it's worth it. "I don't know how they do it. Then there's the talented young baseball player, or say great piano player who is persuaded by parents or friends or orthodox schooling to get into something more lucrative, a more practical trade. You've talked about this before, how sometimes creativity or things people have a passion for are given consideration last."

"Yeah. It's like telling someone to give up their dreams. I realize you can't live off of dreams entirely, but we sure need our dreams and goals too, especially in this world. I think people do have to be careful though. Dreams are okay, but only if someone perseveres and does the foundation work necessary to make them come true." Clara reached for his hand.

"Exactly. That's why I have to start that paramedic course and my photography again, too. I haven't taken any pictures in about six months. This teaching job for the Red Cross is rewarding, but it's not enough. I'm beginning to feel like I'm in too much of a routine, too unchallenged. I need something to break that."

"Your dark room's waiting for you right downstairs." Clara smiled. "And you'll be buried in medical books pretty soon. The holidays are coming up in a few months; let's make a pact to do something over Thanksgiving and Christmas. I'll get back to my poetry and you can work on taking some unique photos and your studies."

He glanced at his wristwatch and realized it was time to get started with dinner. "What do you think about some dinner? We've had good conversation, now let's have some appetizing food." He sat up. "What do you think?"

"I think I'll be waiting for an artistic photo for the living room, and yes, I'm hungry. What do we need? Matches, water. What else?" They both helped each other to a standing position. Bret rubbed his butt and moaned while Clara laughed about it. Then she kissed him on the cheek.

He decided to dig out the pans, dishes and other stuff from his backpack while Clara found the matches and set the small cooler of food near the campfire site.

"Great," Bret said as Clara handed him the matches. "I'll see if I can get what I need and get this thing started. Will you run and get some water? I rinsed out my stinky shirt with that other and this one's almost empty too."

"Sure." She picked up the jug.

"Be careful," he reminded her due to the incident with the bee earlier.

He rearranged the ashy, remaining logs and pile of thinner kindling they had gathered. He placed a fire starter log and some newspaper in the center and with the first match was successful. A few of the stones had gotten displaced, outside the circle, so he carefully replaced them to contain the fire. He dug out the battery operated tape player and decided to set the outdoor mood with some Fleetwood Mac. He thought about Bruce Springsteen or Mellencamp, but changed his mind, considering the serene, Rocky Mountain nature setting. Just like fishing, he thought to himself, don't want to disturb or scare away the wild animals. "Like I said," he mumbled, "it's their home, not ours."

CHAPTER 16

The next thing you're going to learn about old Henry here, is that I'm tired. Tired of fightin' it, tired of trying to break through the iron wall of skepticism. I won't deny that some humans, not the majority, may use allergies as a waste-basket diagnosis, occasionally, for their multitude of physical, psycho-social, and spiritual problems. And I wouldn't be surprised if somewhere along the line, the plea of an allergic disease has been or will be used as a scapegoat, to excuse some type of criminal behavior.

The point I'm trying diligently and honestly to make, by telling my story, is that there are millions, literally millions, of legitimate allergy and asthma-stricken people out there. In fact, asthmatics continue to die each year, because of poor education or management of their very real killer disease.

Now it's true with allergies, there's not always an immune connection. Sometimes it is actually an intolerance or an idiosyncrasy of some sort toward specific irritants or substances, or say the asthmatic system's reaction to proteins or inefficient enzymes, just some of the things I kept trying to get across, like overreacting to harmless things, but nobody would listen.

But believe me, they're out there, struggling along. I'm talking about the bodies that go haywire day after day, the uncontrolled cases, the disagreeable kid who's doped up with the meds by age six, and still feels like a zombie. There's the child who lies down on the floor and starts kicking and crying five minutes after eating a banana or some peanuts. That describes Arnie, another case, a bright, but tortured little boy. I worked with him for years. Finally his mom and dad took him to a board certified allergist. With his allergies managed, he became a healthy, thriving youngster, and his future was saved. Same thing with that other kid, you know, that miracle dust mite case.

I'd like to see a person who thinks allergies or asthma is nothing but a figment of a weak imagination, explain the deaths of people I've worked with, like Marin, or the ones I've heard or read about—horrible, sad, unnecessary deaths.

People who died frightening, tragic deaths because of their allergic or asthmatic nature, cases that involved infants and two year olds, teenagers and adults. The skeptic can work my job for a while, any day. I wish I could be human just for a day, or if I could figure out some miracle of a way to get my story into the hands of humans, I'd say, "Look, here I am. My name is Henry, I'm an antibody, and I'm very real. What does real mean? It means I exist. And if I exist, then my negative parallel also exists, the relentless antigen. Yes sir, I'd say, I'm an antibody and there really is a war going on inside hypersensitive individuals." Then, I'd show them a video of some of the wars, as well as casualties, that have occurred. I'd convince them, once and for all.

Even some of the expert psychologists who damaged victims further by professing that someone should have total control over their health, their fates. Imagine a psychologist telling an asthmatic who grew up trying to survive attacks in a smoke-filled household or a vulnerable individual seriously allergic to peanuts that all of her problems are emotionally based. That just facing her worst fears will make everything all right. Again, the reckless misconception that allergies are all in a person's head, not in a hypersensitive immune system's body!

Work my job, they'd see just how real we are, both of us, antibodies and antigens. Sometimes, when victims died, overuse of medication, or the lack of it caused the final outcome. But so often, no matter how much sincere effort and emergency medical attention the unfortunate patient received after the fact, it was too late, the body was already too far gone, and just wouldn't respond. Same thing with all of the anaphylactic cases, like Marin and Clara, almost. Those darn, rotten allergies. I don't want to burn anybody's ears with four letter curse words, rather than using darn, but I sure feel like it sometimes.

And I'm well aware that the individual has a responsibility to do all he/she can to keep the body's resistance level at a maximum. They can tell me that humans have emotions that tie in, I can buy that. But how is an infant, or a two or four year or ten year old going to have such a tough time with emotions, that it causes such a fatal, immune reaction? It makes me sick to think about the misconceptions regarding allergies and asthma, and the warmongers, my own species, the ones who won't pull back before it's too late.

If there's one thing I've learned, because of Clara and Marin, especially, it's the realization that at some point in time, an antibody must stop merely reacting and take fate into his or her own hands. That's where I *do* believe in the possibility of control. When education is maximized and understanding is accurate, and when everything possible is being done to prevent unnecessary, out of control, suffering; that's the high point I'd like to see the human race achieve, as well as antigens and antibodies.

In hindsight, the only thing that really could have saved Marin is some sort of preventative measures or an adrenaline kit on hand, like Clara had. The saddest part about this a story is that so much of the misery and damage caused by allergies and asthma can be prevented by simply implementing health education and increasing understanding in these areas.

I've seen the agony that the antigen/antibody wars cause, I've tried to fight it, but I think I really need a break. I guess you could say I'm an antibody with limitations. One night last week, I sat wondering if the ones who do die are actually the lucky ones, because the long-lasting physical and mental torture that many of the living ones are subjected to, frankly, just doesn't seem like it's worth it. Think about it. Doesn't the quality of a person's life mean anything? Especially the crippled ones, or the ones who have lost all signs of hope, or in essence, the ones who are physically here, but have died a thousand or more humiliating or emotional deaths. Probably even came close to physical death many times.

But I abandoned the dismal notion almost as quickly as I thought of it, because deep down I happen to be one of those eternal optimists. Where there's a living, breathing, albeit struggling, human being, there's hope. I've seen enough courageous survivors on respirators to know this. That means that I'm somebody who could never forsake the idea of hope.

But then I have friends who tell me, "Never say never," because nobody knows what will happen in a lifetime. That always gets me to thinking about the what-ifs, since I have witnessed a lot of human suffering, not to mention the anguish amidst my fellow antibodies.

So I decided to hang onto the notion that if I ever do feel sort of fatalistically tired, then I can still hang onto hope. The hope that ultimately good forces, rather than evil ones and positive solutions rather than negative ones will empower me to defy my darkest days the wrong to claim "victory."

CHAPTER 17

You're probably anxious to hear what happened to Clara. She did live. But believe me, she was only a matter of seconds from joining all of the other statistics. Just a few allergy facts first.

Individuals allergic to stings of Hymenopterous insects (bees, wasps, etc.) must be treated immediately to prevent a possible fatal outcome. The end can come very suddenly. In most cases, it happens within less than an hour, sometimes within minutes. Bee venom has immediate histaminic effects, but luckily, thank God, Clara and Bret were educated and conscientious enough to have an emergency kit on hand for the treatment of allergic reactions.

It took the quick-acting injection of epinephrine to stabilize her until the Flight for Life helicopter arrived and the flight nurse and paramedic took over. They administered high flow oxygen with a non-rebreather mask. Luckily, the laryngeal edema was under control, so a tracheotomy was avoided. That's when they have to cut into the trachea (windpipe) without delay, to keep the victim breathing.

Bret performed well, as usual, in an emergency situation and simply did whatever he could and had to do, reflexively. But never before had he been so frightened, or witnessed the consequences of anaphylactic shock, a deadly allergic reaction which was about to kill his wife. George, Major Borline, Privates Richey and Porter, Sergeant Birlly, myself, and quite a few of the others, including two apologetic antigen converts, Karin and Ronnie—we all realized what was going on.

It was the same sad story again, we couldn't get the rest of them (the antibodies) to pull back after things were under control. Of course, they refused to listen. Once the lead attackers, broke through the border defenses, most of our reactors just went berserk. We tried to keep the inside perimeter intact, the outside from infiltrating, but fights broke out everywhere. Clara's whole body immediately turned into a battlefield, all out war with some of the neutrophils attacking, once the command was given. And then it went on and on until they began to go crazy attacking everything in sight, including many of Clara's own cells.

George and I said our goodbyes, got things off our chest, and did what any antibody in that predicament does, prepared to die. But converts and Bret saved us and Clara. Thank God. I think I'm the one who's in shock right now.

To the best of my recollection, it happened like this. The mood that afternoon at the campsite was one of serenity and light-heartedness. The smell of barbecued burgers still lingers upon my memory, like a lot of other things that day. The way Bret and Clara joked with each other until they both had side-aches from laughing so hard, then how their mood shifted suddenly to a sentimental one.

We sat in the shade and felt the most comforting breeze, and the quietness of the outdoors. You know, the kind of day that you wish would last forever. They were ready to taste their barbecued dinner when tragedy struck. I remember Bret saying, "Wait for me, wait for me."

"I'm waiting sweetheart, but it's all ready, c'mon, let's eat." Clara gestured with her hands.

"Okay, almost ready, just let me get the salt out of my backpack." He hurried over toward his gear.

When Clara reached out to pick up a can of grape soda, she heard a loud buzzing sound. It startled her. As soon as she made contact, she felt a sharp stinging sensation to her right index finger, looked over, saw a yellow jacket, and screamed. "Bret, help!" she yelled desperately. "I've been stung." That's when Bret proceeded to save our lives.

"Oh God, a bee. What happened? Where's the kit?" Clara recognized the fear and sense of urgency which Bret displayed.

"In my backpack. Hurry Bret! I'm scared." She lifted her index finger to show him the sting.

"Oh no. It's red already and swelling. We know what to do, Clara. Don't worry. I'll get the injection." Then he looked at Clara and his controlled demeanor turned to fear. Her color had changed, and she wheezed and gasped for air. Bret grabbed her shoulders and tried to assist her to a more comfortable sitting position against the tree with the picnic blanket behind her back.

But Clara shouted, "No, just get the kit. I won't be able to breathe. Hurry Bret, in the thigh! In the thigh! I don't want to die."

"I'll do it honey. Hang on." He ran over to the backpack, unzipped the side pouch and grabbed the cellular phone and a pamphlet which had the telephone number to the nearby stables. He then unzipped the other portion of the backpack, tossed out some clothes and found the metal box he needed.

"I got it! I got it!" He raced back and knelt down, expecting Clara to respond. But at that moment, lying on the ground, she gasped again for air, clutched her throat, and pleaded with her eyes for Bret to save her. Then suddenly her eyes closed. She became unconscious and lifeless like a cold corpse. Clara's face and extremities exhibited marked swelling. Cyanosis of the lips had begun to set in.

Bret frantically unclasped the first aid kit and flung it open. He glanced at everything; then picked up a syringe wrapped in cellophane. He tore off the wrapper, looked toward the sky and said, "Please God, please, help me save her." He quickly tore the cap from the syringe and jabbed the needle directly into Clara's right thigh. Although the sharp needle had released the epinephrine into her system, she remained silent and motionless for a few more minutes. Bret checked for a pulse and began respirations, hoping that as soon as the drug kicked in, the airway would open up.

Believe me, I've worked in the field long enough to know that she was a goner without that injection. Deadly chaos had broken loose inside of her. War is such a horror, even for someone who has fought thousands of battles.

Her blood thickened, fluid filled her lungs. I raced over to her heart, and sure enough, it was slowing down and she was on the verge of convulsions due to the lack of blood and oxygen to her brain.

IgE troops had activated the enzymes; then the mast cell granules began to overreact to the bee's venom by releasing histamine and other biochemical warfare. Of course, all of my buddies were doing their jobs. Antibodies make very conscientious soldiers. Like I said, it was impossible to get through to many of them and change their thinking. They were trained, conditioned to react a certain way, but the good that evolved from this unfortunate incident is the fact that I did manage to pull, like I said, some fellow comrades out of the darkness, and even, believe it or not, those two antigens. Maybe they couldn't sign on as antibodies, but they could sure quit their jobs as terrorizing antigens, and perhaps become educators in the field.

Many had finally figured it out; how we can be so destructive ourselves, rather than preserving and protecting and even to the point of fatal overreactions. It never made any sense in this line of work. Try to counterattack and do some good, and look what can happen. I figure it's all a matter of balance, finding that immunological equilibrium.

I handed them all my sob story about Marin, how we lost her. That's what did it and the close call with Clara. Then I played the Army Sergeant role, made sure the granules did their job, but then proceeded to beg them all to help me prevent the fatal reaction. You see, we are the good guys, but the sad truth is that we can be as dangerous as we are helpful. The antigen troops are the bad guys, the relentless antagonists, but there are ways to fight them and win.

Clara won, thanks to an antidote that was on hand and administered properly, and a follow-up emergency rescue. Every time I hear a helicopter whirling by in the air these days, I think of that huge yellow and orange monster of a chopper that descended from the clear blue and transported Clara on what certainly could have been a "flight for life."

The shot stabilized her, but who knows if she was out of the woods yet. That close to death and you don't want to take any chances. Bret was lucky he could get through to the horse stable so they could call 911 and dispatch the hospital helicopter. The medics got as close as they could to us. That was another problem, transporting, by foot, Clara on the spine board to the helicopter location. I can still hear the sound of the engines and the chopper blades swirling around on take off and the pilot shouting, "Air Rescue One to dispatcher, we're in the air now and have the stable post-anaphylactic patient on board."

I noticed the dedicated look in the flight nurse's face as she adjusted the liter valve on the oxygen. What a close call, I thought to myself. I'm getting too old for this kind of adventure.

CHAPTER 18

So that's it. That's my story, and I suppose if you're an antibody, or if anyone in your family, yourself, or your friends have ever had any experiences with allergies or asthma, or maybe if you study this stuff or if you work in the field, you'll find it interesting. If not, that's your choice. All I know is, it's not my problem anymore. I've done my job, and what I felt I had to do. After all, who else could have told you the inside story?

George and I are checking on some sources, see if we can get transferred to some controlled, mild case down south near the beaches or something. And it's going to be with someone who wears one of those bracelets and carries an emergency kit, especially an epipen, just in case. We're getting too old for this kind of drama in our lives. Clara knows how to take care of herself, and some specialist troops took over since a bunch of the others were wiped out, so she'll be fine.

It's time for me to take some time out for living, not in fear, not in frustration, not in anger or pain, not misunderstood, not playing "hero," and certainly not chained to the past. One other thing that George and I found comfort in during our ordeal with the ones we lost, or others who encountered very close brushes with death, was the ability to accept the fact that sometimes an antibody does what he/she has to do, not what he/she wants to do. It took us both a long time to learn that. You know what I'd like though, most of all? To be myself. I just want to be Henry, all masks and pretensions removed. I feel whole again, and free, really free. At last.

Although a clergybody once told me that, "In actuality, commitment is the truest kind of freedom." Maybe I'll feel like an old goatbody out to pasture. The field of allergy and immunology is all I really know. But I also know, within my heart, that it's time to let go.

One final thought. If I had the chance to tell allergic victims one thing, I'd tell them that: bodies, minds, and spirits that try hard to heal themselves, against all odds, no matter how sick, disillusioned, or handicapped, no matter how long it might take—they're the real heroes.

A poet, Kay Kaye, once wrote, "Survivors are among us: from concentration camps, tragedies, sickness, from the dungeons of neglect and abuse. But only for a short time in their lives were they 'victims,' because from very early on, they began surviving or else they wouldn't still be here."

What it comes down to in the final analysis is that nobody can bring you peace but yourself. I'd try to convince hypersensitive individuals to exercise an indomitable will and personal responsibility, as much as possible, so that they wouldn't have to feel helpless or hopeless, or overwhelmed by threatening external conditions. The body's state of immunity and equilibrium will continuously be challenged throughout a sufferer's lifetime.

However, the individual's state of mind and willingness to learn about and work toward the possibilities for better health will play such an important part in determining his or her quality of life.

Like Frankl, one of the human heroes I've read about, he could not and did not deny the concentration camp's existence and suffering which he endured. But, he did manage to rely on his most self-transcendent capabilities to deny the limitations of a specific detrimental environment and set of circumstances. Nothing, absolutely nothing, could take away or destroy his will to live and right to enjoy life, and hope and dream for a happier, healthier, freer tomorrow. Same thing with the survivors I've been reading about in the paper lately, some innocent people sitting in prisons who, according to actual facts and evidence, have proven their innocence. But it seems, nobody will listen. I can't imagine whole families, years destroyed, because of actual crimes against innocent people, or some distortion of justice. And yet they survive, just like Frankl, somehow.

Finally, in regards to my fellow antibodies and the allergic/asthmatic population, I'd wish them all good luck. "The best of luck to you," from Henry. I conveyed the same sentiments to my buddy George one day.

"Say, Henry, tell them I said good luck too."

"Folks, George wishes everyone good luck too."

"You know Henry, the boss just handed me a scoop about a case out west, in California, lots of sunshine and sandy beaches, just what we wanted."

"Well, what are we waiting for?" I asked excitedly.

"Okay, let's go. There is one thing though. It seems we've been promoted to research, for the big one, AIDS. Now don't get touchy, let me expla...."

But George didn't get the chance to finish. He knew by the look on my face that I didn't want any part of it.

"Oh no you don't," I frowned and shook my head fervently. "There are two diseases that I flatly refuse to work on. You know how I feel about AIDS and cancer. Allergies and asthma are discouraging enough sometimes."

I knew progress was being made in the two fields, but cancer hit close to home, too many relatives or favorite people lost to it, and AIDS, all I could remember were the years I spent with Ryan, a young kid who eventually lost his brave battle. He was a real trooper. All I said was, "Sure George, remember Ryan, all those years of fighting, then we lost him. I'm not going through that again."

My dazed expression must have been apparent to him.

"Henry, Henry! Are you listening?" He shouted. "This is different, Henry, believe me. We'll be working with some specialists, MABS (monoclonal antibodies).

Immunotherapy is finally recognized as a crucial modality. They're listening to us Henry, understand?"

"Mono what?' I backtracked. Usually *I* was the one trying to teach George something.

"Oh let me explain it to you later. Just say you'll think about it," George pleaded. "We're a team pal. I need you. We can do some good."

After a few moments of serious contemplation, all of my mental barriers for refusing George's suggestions dissipated. Actually, I felt kind of relieved, to tell you the truth. It's a strange thing about living, seems to be much more worthwhile and exciting when there's purpose and direction involved. "How old did you say this case was?" I asked.

"Only 27, and you know there's a lot of hope at that age, especially with all of this new research, and of course all of our experience, and this lady, I promise, she's a fighter Henry," he rambled on eagerly. They're coming up with all kinds of new, exciting things to try. Epipens are getting better and better all the time, too. We just have to get people to carry them. Just like you say, keep trying to get through to the antibody over-reactors *and* the humans. I'm telling you buddy, it's a good thing we're both on our way to retirement, because, just like that other doctor in Chicago, trying to wipe out all of the IgE battalions, we might be on our way out, as far as the field of allergy and asthma goes."

Here we go again, I thought. George and his big dreams. But he's right. Yes indeed, understanding allergy and immunology will lead humankind to many answers and much healing someday, if humans and antibodies will just listen.

"Yes, indeed, it sure will. Allergies and..."

"It sure will what? What Clara, what are you mumbling about?" Bret loudly requested an answer while he shook Clara's right arm.

"Hmm? What? No. No. Leave me alone. I wanna sleep some more. I don't want to leave this dream yet." Clara rolled over, ignoring her inquisitive husband.

"What dream Clara?" What sure will? What about allergies?" he persisted.

Clara rubbed her eyes, rolled back on her left side, faced Bret and explained in a shortcut manner. "It's a long, incredible story honey. I'll tell you all about it later, okay? Right now, I'm tired and I want to sleep in. It was all about this little character, Henry. He was, I mean I guess I was, an antibody inside people's bodies, you know, like that movie, *Fantastic Voyage*. God, I remember all this fighting between the allergies and us, the antibodies. It was awful."

"You've been reading too much of that book, *The Body is the Hero*. Who is that by? Glasser?"

"Yeah, Doctor Glasser. Hey, by the way, thanks for saving my life last night. You saved me. We were hiking, just like we did last weekend, but this time I got stung by that yellow jacket we saw, then went into anaphylactic shock, and you and the Flight for Life nurse and paramedic rescued me. That was the weird part. One minute I felt like myself, but then, well you know how dreams jump around and don't make sense all the time, all of a sudden, I'd become Henry and I was inside of my body fighting the antigens, literally fighting them with my friend George. He was another antibody. Oh shoot, George isn't real, darn, I'm gonna miss him."

"You're right, go back to sleep."

"But I'm awake now. So you get to listen to the whole story. You see, it all started with this girl Marin..."

"Oh no you don't," Bret jumped out of bed. "Not without my coffee."

"All right, all right. But hurry back. Henry and I will be waiting for you."

Two cups of coffee later, Bret returned as promised.

"Okay honey, I'm raring to go now. I want to hear more about your night job of being an antibody. What was his name, Henry?"

"Yeah, Henry. I was Henry and I had a friend, George. He sounded just like Walter Matthau when he talked or laughed. We were soldiers and like detectives. I kept talking about all the different cases I'd worked on, allergic and asthmatic victims, similar to ones at the clinic. Most lived, but some of them died. I guess I felt guilty about this one girl named Marin that my friends and I had killed, because of an antigen-antibody war. So I must have been telling the story from Henry's perspective and it seemed so real."

"Hmm. Well I'm curious, what's an antibody look like?"

"Well, seemed like I was shaped like the letter Y and, oh yeah, it was funny. We both had on these blue tennis shoes and George had bigger feet than I did. Strangest thing though, it was like we were a real army, but all I saw us wearing was more like a basketball shirt or something."

"What? That's funny. I'm trying to picture you, a tiny little creature, shaped like a Y with blue tennies. Hey, wait a minute. I just read something the other day about antibodies. You say you kept going from case to case. Were these guys old or young, I mean you and George? Because, as you probably know, antibodies don't live a long time and it said something about when the host dies so does the antibody." He said it smartly, as if he had just been promoted to genius. "So there you go, major flaw in you dream. Henry or you couldn't have gone from case to case because if that girl died, then..."

"I cannot absolutely believe this! I'm telling you that I experienced the most incredibly vivid, cartoon-like, yet seemingly realistic fantastic voyage through human bodies last night, actually watched and felt what it was like to witness an all out war between antigens and antibodies and you sit here talking about medical correctness. That's like talking syntax to Thoreau or Mark Twain. IT WAS A DREAM DEAR. Remember? Anything can happen in a dream! It doesn't have to make perfect sense. Don't ever go absolutely practical on me, okay? I couldn't stand it."

Bret joked around, puckered his bottom lip and pretended to hold his head down in shame. "Sorry."

"Forgiven. Now let me tell you the rest of the story. Just try to pretend you're a kid or something. Dispense with the grown-up critiquing, just for an hour or so."

"Got it, understood. Go for it Clara. Tell me all about your adventure." He put his arm around her and she started again, from the beginning.

"Well, like I said, there was this girl, Marin...."

EPILOGUE

A WHOLE NEW CHAPTER
IN MY LIFE

Every allergic and asthmatic child in the world dreams. Mostly, the ultimate dream is to be able to breathe normally and to run and play like other kids. I, at age sixty now, consider myself one of the luckiest allergic/asthmatics who ever lived. I really do. Why? Because I got lucky. Oh, I worked hard at it too, believe me. But I got lucky— survived and escaped the dungeon of sickness. Not only that, year after year, like the free-spirited bird, Jonathan Livingston Seagull, I soared, and chose to keep right on flying until I broke through even more, seemingly impossible, barriers and flew right into the highest realms of wellness.

Whenever someone is healthy, more dreams can come to realization, so I kept living life, enjoying a loving relationship, attending college, working as a nurse, writing, and became a published author. Much of what you read throughout Henry's case assignments is how my crazy and wild antibodies affected me for much of my life. But it's not the whole story, therefore the epilogue.

Millions of allergic/asthmatic kids are lucky if they can ever even have a cat or dog. I've had pets all my life. Every aspect of any sick child's life is always affected. So why is it that I kept going to school and learning, even though I had plenty of sick days and lips puffed up with the ugliest cold sores a person ever did see?

Why was I able to swim at Lake Robinson, the manmade lake I loved so much as a child? Why did I keep on running and wheezing and surviving potentially fatal asthma attacks? Because I wanted to join in the fun and play: baseball, softball, tag football, basketball, cricket, red light-green light, kick the can and ride my bike! In the wintertime, I went ice skating, and sledding. I didn't want to be different, although I was. But, why me? Why and how did I survive? One more breath at a time, I guess. One breath at a time.

I spent a lot of days and nights struggling to breathe, hanging in there, just so I could have one more day of life. I never gave up. And look where it got me. I can't believe it. Sixty years of life. To me, it is a true miracle. Not only that, but I believe wholeheartedly that it is a miracle that any allergic/asthmatic kid can achieve. Will it be easy? Nope. Just living life with ups and downs is not easy. Add to it these two hypersensitive immune system afflictions—allergies and asthma—and it gets really tough much of the time. Possible to endure, participate in life, achieve and enjoy though? Absolutely!

Some of my earliest memories of being frightened to death, struggling to breathe and fighting for my life are at my grandmother's house in Kingsford Heights. All I had was Vick's Vapor Rub on my neck and chest to try and ease the medical crisis situation. The thing is, with any one of those early attacks, at my grandma's house or at home, I could have easily died. Throughout my lifetime, believe me, so many times due to severe asthma attacks, I could have died.

Neither my early autobiography about surviving a crazy, out of control immune system or *Sneezing Seasons* is the end of the story. Allergies and asthma are only the tips of the devastating iceberg when it comes to problems related to a hypersensitive immune system. Thus, this epilogue, brings to light the next chapter in my life—the terror of an autoimmune affliction and a couple of poems that prove I, once again, counterattacked and lived a miraculous-like life at times.

That's right. Things got worse. At age forty-eight while working as a nurse, I contracted Strep throat. A few weeks later, I was fighting for my life. Actually, I've never stopped fighting for quality of life, ever since then. Little did I know a hypersensitive immune system could go even more haywire, start attacking healthy cells to the point of no return, if not counterattacked. So that's what I did, started fighting back. That's a whole other story, a follow-up time in my life and book titled: *Autoimmunity Counterattack: A Sequel/The Healthy Road Back.* (Non-profit.) It's "the rest of the story," as Paul Harvey often quipped.

After two years of being critically ill off and on, I got better. Again, one of the lucky ones, I was able to go back to work and participate and enjoy life again. Two years of chronic pain and crippling symptoms certainly derailed my life, but at age fifty, I was in the midst of a comeback. So much so, I knew I needed to celebrate big-time! After all, I truly never thought I'd live to see my fiftieth birthday.

What a way to rejoice! It was my second bicycle tour actually—this one, an adventure on two wheels across the United States. There were twelve of us. We named ourselves, "The Dirty Dozen." I considered my riding comrades my guardian angels. We began in beautiful San Diego, California and finalized our tour by dipping our worn tires in the Atlantic Ocean in St. Augustine, Florida. Just another miracle to me.

Now for those poetic literary rides. C'mon, join me, let's hop on Dream Drive!

PREVIEW

AUTOIMMUNITY COUNTERATTACK: A SEQUEL/THE HEALTHY ROAD BACK!

(Note: Partial contents from foreword and book with some revisions)

FROM THE FOREWORD

By Dr. Katherine M. Poehlmann, Ph.D/RA Survivor

Just as on a cycling trip, the scenery varies as you read this book. You will discover the author's personal health history and startling statistics about autoimmune conditions such as: rheumatoid arthritis and lupus. Within the book are evocative poems, and appeals for sectors of society (medical, political, research, media, grassroots groups, schools, celebrities, and corporations) to pool their resources and talents in a united effort to solve the autoimmunity puzzle.

Galvan has an uplifting story to tell and an important message to deliver. I am honored to write the foreword to this book because I have personally experienced the same frustrations in trying to find answers to my debilitating RA conditions. *The road to wellness at this point in medical history should be straight and clearly marked with helpful signposts. Sadly, it is not.*

There should now, in this 21st century, be widespread consensus that autoimmune disorders and hypersensitivity are genuine, painful, debilitating conditions. Each year, a growing number of patients are afflicted, many of them children. Yet patients are told they are malingering or being hypochondriacs because they do not appear to have observable and measurable symptoms. They are given simplistic advice to "just eat right and reduce stress" and sent on their way. They are not given specific diagnostic tests that could shed some light on the problem(s). Perhaps, most importantly, from a psychological standpoint, they are denied a sincere appreciation and acknowledgment of the very real pain they feel. (1)

Kind Regards,
Katherine M. Poehlmann, Ph.D. (April 12, 2005)

"All the magnificence of our immune system can be turned against the body and cause disease. It now appears that those early whisperers were right. The immune system, always the counter attacker, sometimes it misreads the signs and launches itself at our cells just as relentlessly as it would any foreign invader. (2)

The Body is the Hero
Dr. Ronald J. Glasser

"Antibody soldiers patrol, defend, and protect human bodies. When well-intended (but misguided) or rebel over-reactive antibodies terrorize and cause an immune system to become a person's own worst enemy—all one can do is hope, pray, and counterattack." (3)

Autoimmunity Counterattack:
A Sequel/The Healthy Road Back
Gail Galvan

DREAM DRIVE

ADVENTURE ROLL CALL

Bicycles, feet, minds
set to motion. Waves goodbye
to the Pacific Ocean.
Florida bound, a coast away.
Eager to pedal, day by day.
Arizona's desert sun, sandy dunes,
challenging, adventurous rides.
Lagoon saloons.
Jukebox Diamond sings us songs.
"Biker" bars, "Hey, we belong!"
Moonlit skies blanket us at night.
Day breaks and we tour the sights.
Roll call first.
Get ready to ride.
The day's planned out,
nothing left to decide.
Schwinn, Raleigh, Peugeot and Captain Co-Motion.
"Start rolling. Be careful. Use lots of suntan lotion."
Cannondale, Nishiki,
and that long shot, Black Beauty,
"Gear up, head out, you're on tonight
for dinner duty."
Ti-Tiger, Sequoia, no hurry.
Speed masters, we know.
Good leaders, leisurely ride-on,
eastbound we go.
Off to see the states,
to ride with the dream-winds.
"Check all panniers and brake shoes,
then saddle in."
Roll call, we can't forget
Trek and Trek.
Will they be riding neck to neck?

Explorers, cowboys and Indians,
how the west was won.
Historical landmarks,
more long stretches, scorching sun.
Studying birds and cactus, diversified.
Animals, armadillos, snakes, tarantulas,
spotted roadside.
Ah, here he comes, roll call,
that green limousine, one of a kind.
His country flag, flying high all the time.
An Aussie named Gary.
Like all the rest, cycles hard all day.
In the eve, loves to tarry.
So here we are,
touring by bike, not car.
America so beautiful, so free.
Riding on, until it's Florida we see.

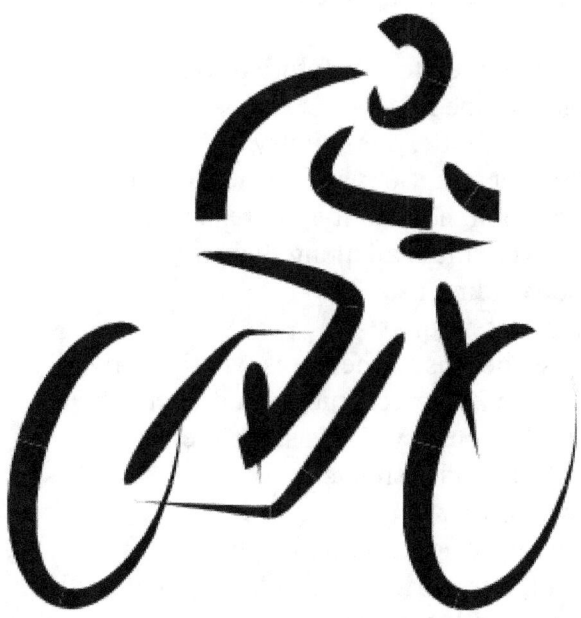

HIGHLIGHTS OF A ROAD TRIP

(Dedicated to eleven amazing adventure cyclists and the
Adventure Cycling Association in Missoula, Montana)

Fascination across the U.S.A.
Here are some highlights. Right this way.
San Diego sunshine. Adult cyclists at play.
The beach and dream that beckoned us.
Hills, mountains, rivers and lakes,
bridges to marvel at and cross.
Snakes and tarantulas at our feet.
Caterpillars on the move.
Even they reach their destination.
California dreamin' again and again.
Riding with the wind, we ride.
Desert sun, desert wildlife, stickers sabotage.
Thorns in our dream-tires. Sunshine so hot.
Burn, cyclist, burn.
Railroad history, expressed to this future of ours.
Not horses, bikes, we ride in cars.
Black Jack Newman, Globe, our country.
The history, Billy, that kid. So many stories to tell.
Silver city, Silver Moon, hospitality galore, so kind.
Mascots too, they were there all along the way,
welcoming us, befriending us,
the temporary homeless tourist.
Yet never homeless, because America is where we live.
Bike shop magic. The Zen mechanics of a dream vehicle.
"Laundry, last call for laundry! Let's share the load."
"Map meeting!" Tour leader shouts.
"Let's plan out which way to go."
Indian villages and historical markers from west to east.
The history of it all, our world, our forefathers and mothers,
Indians, explorers and adventurers like ourselves.

Gila forests, cave dwellings
From the primitive days of yore.
Zippers at night because we camped.
Night sounds of a natural world out there under the stars.
American peace pipe stories, along with the tragedies,
the dark side—unpleasantries of our history. No escape.
Oldies in cadence, music to travel to.
Soothing to aching feet. We ride, mile after mile,
town after town, we ride.
State to state signs mean so much.
Crossing over, one quick, special touch.
Shady spots, thirst-quenchers,
Ode to the cactus again and again.
We love our homeland where wild cactus grows
and buffalo still roam. River crossings, deer crossings.
They jumped right out in front of me!
Texas barbeque and the perfect host.
We'll be back to toast you and the others,
I'm sure. Someday, the return.
We'll be seeing you in our dreams.
Texas trail, Texas trail, we follow our ancestors.
Harley high-fives, low-fives (It's a biker thing).
Biker buddies out there on the road.
Cravings, we stop. The search is on.
Sushi! Waffle house! Taco Bell! Pizza!
Ice cream shop. Stop!
Extremes. Seminole sunrise one day in the life of a tourist,
jets overhead the next. We travel on. We ride.
Biker wagon trains of today.
Well-wagons capture the essence,
the passion for wellness and adventure.
Taps, music bonds us just like Neil Diamond did.
We rock into the El Paso nightlife.
Apaches, more legends. The Indians still live.
They are our neighbors.
Side trips taken by those two characters.

They had to see the Alamo.
Reunited for Baxter's delicious night out
and musical dessert.
Extremes in New Orleans. Way down.
Jazzy city, dazzling lights, saxophone jazz.
Homeless kids on the streets of America.
Library Lit Fest. Watched a yarn spinner spin stories.
Felt the creative fire within from a Hip-Hop Tyree author.
Sat mesmerized by a Caribbean Calabash wonder
and got inspired by an Olympia version
of a star-lit success story.
Closer to the east coast, we ride. Southern comforts,
Cajun country, Cajun cooking.
Louisiana purchase of a soda pop.
Remembering Daniel Boone and Davy Crockett.
They were good men. Miles to go. We ride.
The days are long, but we ride.
The road is long, but we ride and love to ride.
The outdoors is ours to breathe in.
From American fast foods to dining extravaganzas,
we re-energize. Mental counteractions
for tired tourists in motion.
Cool swims and calm nights. We sleep, we rise, we ride.
Silly socks, time to buy silly socks.
From state to state, silly socks.
The mountains are behind us. State signs, one after another.
We cross over. Alas, before our eyes, destination.
Florida is real.
We hug. Finally, sand in our toes again.
We dip our worn tires in an Atlantic Ocean wonder.
Our dream comes true. St. Augustine, alas,
You welcome us.
Like all the rest from the Wild West.
Explorers of yesterday.
Bicycling, the modern way back to the saddle.
This modern day wagon train that came your way.

Happy day! Oh happy day!
Sightseeing and celebrations, again we're at play.
The healthy mountaintop memories belong to us.
What's this? Oh no. The top of this mountain,
it's just the bottom, a new beginning
of another mountain to climb.
Adventurers, our traveling is never done.

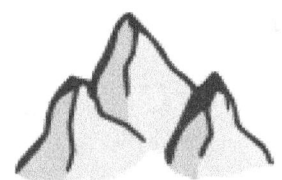

MAGICAL MOMENT

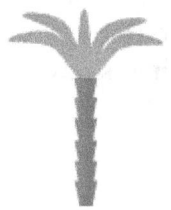

"As I ponder here
at the Florida coastline,
the sign of the cross
in pantomime—
Thanks be to God
and all the rest
who played a part
in helping me live
this destiny dream,
so impassioned,
within my heart."

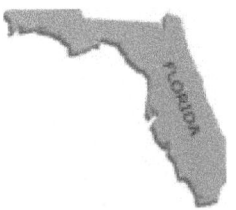

Eternal thanks, Adventure Cyclist/Southern Tier, 2003
Allergic/Asthmatic/RA Survivor

EMERGENCY LANE

911: A CALL FOR HELP

AND THE EMERGENCY IS....

EMS: 9-1-1. What is your emergency?

CALLER: Hypersensitive, self-attacking and
         malfunctioning immune systems.

EMS: Where is your location?

CALLER: All over the world, inside human
         bodies.

EMS: When did this happen, is it happening
         right now?

CALLER: It happens every day, minute, and yes,
         it's happening within millions of
         people right now.

EMS: What is your name? Who's calling?

CALLER: My name? My name is not what
         counts. I'm just one of the millions
         who endures hypersensitivity. I could
         be anyone, your significant other, your
         parent, your child, neighbor, teacher—
         trust me, someone you know is
         suffering or dying right now.

EMS: Let me switch you over to my
         supervisor to see what we can do.

CALLER: Thank you.

EMS: Hello, do you have a *specific* emergency?

CALLER: Yes, this is a MEDIC ALERT! Millions are suffering or becoming disabled or dying right now because of hypersensitivity, autoimmunity, even immunodeficiency. This is a call for help, for increased understanding regarding immune system disorders/emergencies. Please help!

EMS: What can we do?

CALLER: Understand the problem. Tell your medics, doctors, nurses, nurses' aides, parents, even teachers. Please understand and help. Thank you!

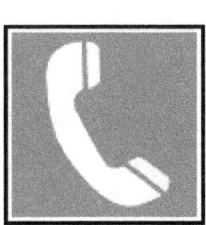 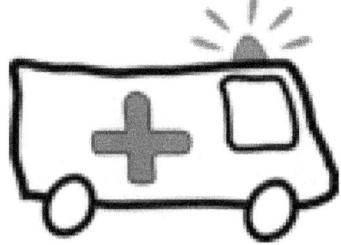

FACTUAL ROADWAYS

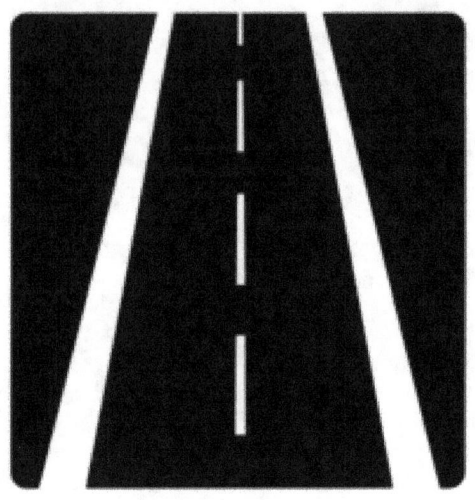

ASTOUNDING FACTS AND FIGURES

FACTS: Statistics vary at times from various sources, but according to the Allergy and Asthma Foundation of America: (4 and 5)

FIFTY MILLION Americans suffer from all types of allergies (1 in 5 Americans).

Allergy prevalence has increased overall since the early 1980's across all ages, genders, and racial groups.

Allergies is the 5th leading chronic disease in the U.S. amongst all ages.

Allergies are the 3rd most common chronic disease amongst children through age 18 years old.

Allergies are the most frequent reported chronic conditions in children—limiting activities for more than 40% of them.

Each year, allergies accounts for more than 17 million outpatient office visits, primarily in spring and fall.

Nearly 400 Americans die each year due to drug allergies from penicillin.

There are more than 200 deaths that occur each year due to food allergies.

Ten deaths each year are due to severe reactions to a latex allergy.

Annual costs due to allergies is estimated at nearly 14.5 billion dollars.

Adult allergies (hay fever) is the 5th leading chronic disease and a major cause of work absenteeism accounting for 4 million missed or lost days each year.

Daily asthma statistics are alarming too:

Nearly twenty-five million Americans suffer from asthma.

Asthma is the most common chronic condition among children.

44,000 asthma attacks occur daily.
36,000 kids miss school daily
27,000 adults miss work daily
4,700 people visit the ER daily
1,200 are admitted to the hospital daily

9 ASTHMATICS DIE DAILY!

FACT: Each year in the month of May, on the first Tuesday, asthma awareness is paid attention to and heightened by World Asthma Day. World-wide asthma takes its heavy toll too. That's one thing about allergic and asthmatic sufferers/survivors, they are never alone in their fight. According to the National Institute of Allergies and Infectious Diseases, world-wide, 230 million people are affected by asthma. (6) As May (National Asthma Awareness month) rolls around each year, I always thank God, good doctors, and meds for all of my healthy comebacks, essentially, for my life. Now, on to that other devastating tip of the hypersensitive disease iceberg— autoimmune afflictions.

FACT: Autoimmune disease refers to a varied group of over 100 chronic illnesses that involve almost every human organ system. It includes diseases of all bodily systems as well as the skin and other connective tissues, eyes, blood, and blood vessels. In all of these diseases, the underlying problem is similar—the body's immune system becomes misdirected, attacking the very organs it was designed to protect. (7)

FACT: Although children and men are also affected at times, autoimmune diseases occur in women about 75% of the time. (8)

FACT: In one study autoimmune diseases were cited in the top ten leading causes of all deaths among U.S. women age 65 and younger. (9)

FACT: These diseases represent the fourth largest cause of disability among women in the United States. (10)

FACT: Autoimmune diseases occur while women often look healthy and because the diseases affect multiple body systems, their symptoms are often misleading, which hinders accurate diagnosis. (11)

FACT: Over 45% of patients with autoimmune diseases have been labeled chronic complainers in the earliest stages of their illnesses. (12)

FACT: Unlike cancer, autoimmunity has not been accepted or labeled as a category of disease. (13)

FACT: The American Autoimmune Related Disease Association recognizes the need for more collaboration in research regarding autoimmunity as the underlying cause of autoimmune related diseases and advocates the use of Diagnostic Centers as a critical need for early diagnosis which may prevent significant and lifelong health problems. (14)

FACT: According to estimates, autoimmune diseases cost $86 billion dollars per year. (15)

FACT: Lupus is a chronic, autoimmune disease which causes inflammation of various parts of the body, especially the skin, joints, blood and kidneys. The immune system normally protects the body against viruses, bacteria, and other foreign materials. In an autoimmune disease like lupus, the immune system loses its ability to tell the difference between foreign substances and its own cells and tissues. The immune system then makes antibodies directed against "self." (16)

FACT: Lupus, an autoimmune disease, is not contagious, cancerous or related to AIDS, the immunodeficiency disease. (17)

FACT: Lupus affects 1 out of every 185 Americans.
(18)

FACT: The average lupus patient has symptoms for 3 to 10 years prior to diagnosis. Lupus is more prevalent in African Americans, Latinos, Native Americans, and Asians. (19)

FACT: Autoimmune diseases range from mild to disabling and potentially life-threatening. Although lupus also ranges from mild to life-threatening, 5,000 Americans die every year, yet the majority of the cases can be controlled with proper treatment. Many lupus deaths can be avoided if the patient is diagnosed early. (20)

FACT: While medical science has not yet developed a method for curing lupus and other autoimmune related afflictions, new research brings unexpected findings and increased hope each year. (21)

FACT: Autoimmune and inflammatory diseases cause considerable suffering. Rheumatoid arthritis, multiple sclerosis, type I diabetes, asthma, and inflammatory bowel disease affect more the one-tenth of all people. This figure is even higher if hardening of the arteries and neurodegenerative diseases are included. The progress of all these diseases includes a distinct inflammatory component. What all these diseases have in common is that they more of less selectively attack the function of vital tissues, organs, even completely destroying them sometimes. These diseases feature imbalances in the regulation of inflammatory and immunologically active cells. (22)

FACT: Rheumatoid arthritis, or RA, is a common form of arthritis. (Arth means joint, itis means inflammation.) RA causes inflammation in the lining of the joints, leading to warmth, decreased range of motion, swelling and pain in the joint. RA tends to persist for many years. Typically, it affects many different joints throughout the body and can cause damage to the cartilage, bone, tendons, and ligaments of the joints. (23)

FACT: Occasionally, people with RA develop inflammation of the linings that surround the heart (pericarditis) and lungs (pleuritis) or inflammation of the lung tissue itself. In some instances, people with RA may develop vasculitis (inflammation of the blood vessels) that can cause inflammation and tissue damage affecting the skin, nerves, and other organs. (24)

FACT: In the United States, almost one percent of the population, or 2.1 million people, has RA. (25)

FACT: Females are 2-3 more times likely to develop RA than males. (26)

FACT: RA does not follow a benign course. It is associated with signs of morbidity, disability and mortality. Daily living activities are impaired in most patients. (27)

FACT: After 5 years of disease (RA), approximately 33% of patients will not be working. After 10 years, approximately half will have substantial functional disability. (28)

FACT: Life expectancy for patients with RA is shortened by 5-10 years, although those who respond to therapy may have lower mortality rates. (29)

FACT: At present, the infection connection with regard to RA remains a controversial issue, although there are many researchers, doctors, and RA sufferers who support the belief that RA is caused by an infection connection. Long term tetracycline antibiotic therapy (preferably started at the first onset of symptoms) has been proposed for years by the late Thomas McPherson Brown and others for RA, as well as for other "connective tissue diseases," such as scleroderma and lupus. (30)

FACT: At present, some physicians will not recommend tetracycline therapy for RA unless prodded by a patient, and some not even then. This choice of medication is far safer than steroids, aspirin, non-steroidal anti-inflammatory agents, gold and methotrexate currently in vogue for the treatment of this chronic and debilitating disease. Although, again, I have read that the antibiotic therapy works best if used early on as first diagnosed. Unfortunately, as the facts state here and I sadly realized, the diagnosis of an autoimmune affliction can take years. (31)

FACT: Thousands of arthritics a year still die from the silent ulcers caused by the use of NSAIDS for management of their symptoms. (32)

FUTURE FAIRWAYS

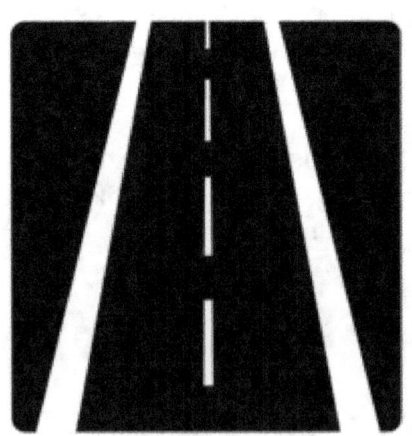

Someday there will be a cure for allergies, asthma, multiple sclerosis, rheumatoid arthritis, Grave's disease, type I immune-mediated diabetes, Chron's disease, strange-sounding afflictions named systemic lupus erythematosus and thrombocytopenic purpura, and many other autoimmune related diseases. Scientists, researchers, healthcare professionals, and many organizations are working diligently to understand the causes and adverse effects of autoimmunity while enabling those afflicted to enjoy an improved quality of life. Health education, prevention, healthy management, when necessary, and especially eradication of disease, disability, and death are goals.

Yet, unlike cancer, which is a well-known category or etiology of disease, autoimmunity, which is responsible for the underlying cause of at least 100 chronic illnesses, remains "among the most poorly understood and poorly recognized of any category of illness." (33) The diseases are often referred to by using lengthy, barely able to pronounce, confusing names.

Millions suffer from autoimmunity, yet when asked what the name of their disease is, sometimes it's very difficult to get the words right, let alone explain how the disease process works. Imagine trying to ramble off a diagnosis of ankylosing spondylitis, eosinophilic granuloma, myasthenia gravis, Hashimoto's thyroiditis, antiphospholid antibody syndrome, systemic lupus erythematosus or a histio (tissue) incompatibility of some sort and expect someone to understand what disease is causing so much misery and threat to quality of life, or to life itself.

Autoimmune related diseases rank high on the priority list of the National Institutes of Health, Office of Research on Women's Health. Some fifty million Americans are afflicted and autoimmunity targets women 75% of the time. Autoimmunity represents the 4th largest cause of disease among women in the U.S., and one study reported that autoimmune diseases made the top ten list of leading causes of all deaths among U.S. women age 65 and younger. (34)

So what is autoimmunity exactly? What is this disease process that is causing so much disability and death? Well, let me introduce you to it, and hopefully increase your understanding of autoimmunity as an etiology of disease, if you are not aware of it.

I've thought about this quite a bit and I think the easiest way to explain autoimmunity, for people who are just learning about autoimmune diseases or for someone who wants to gain a better understanding, is to refer first to the immunization process. Most people understand immunizations, vaccines, at least somewhat, right?

The reason why many life-threatening illnesses no longer pose a threat to the human race is because immunization provides a strong defense against deadly diseases. Vaccines contain a weakened (attenuated) or killed (inactivated) form of disease-causing bacteria or viruses, or components of these microorganisms, that trigger a response by the body's immune system. One of the many things I learned in nursing school.

Talk about adaptation—we need protection from a deadly disease and all we have to do is introduce a little bit of the weakened or dead form of it into our systems and when the fight is on, our body sees it as an enemy, attacks and destroys. "Vaccines stimulate our bodies to make antibodies—proteins that specifically recognize and target the bacteria and viruses against which the vaccines are designed, and that helps eliminate them from the body when we encounter them." (35)

Unfortunately, there are always new bacterial and viral diseases emerging, and it can take years to develop a safe, effective vaccine. If it were a simple process, AIDS (acquired immune deficiency syndrome), other infectious diseases, and even immunologically-caused illnesses might no longer be a threat to us.

In the case of allergies, the immune system reacts and hurries to our defense. An invader threatens us, then our body, equipped with antibodies to the invasive substance, counterattacks. Allergic individuals, unfortunately, must deal with hypersensitive immune systems, and far too often, the immune system overdoes it, reacts to harmless substances, for example: dust, pollen, or certain foods such as peanuts or shrimp.

"The disease-producing mechanisms in autoimmunity are called hypersensitive reactions. Autoimmunity occurs when there is some interruption of the usual control process, allowing lymphocytes to avoid suppression, or when there is an alteration of some body tissue so that it is no longer recognized as self and is thus attacked." (36). This can be disastrous for a person who is afflicted with an autoimmune-related disease.

Maybe an even easier understanding of autoimmunity and other immune system disorders could be conveyed by thinking of immune system control similar to how blood sugar control works. Diabetes is much more understood, in my opinion. So I'm waiting on the cool invention called an immunometer. Check the blood, do whatever a hypersensitive has to do in order to get back to immunological equilibrium. If a body is (hyper) overreacting, blood factors and values show inflammation and chaotic reactions are occurring; then fix it. If it is (hypo) deficient and not reacting enough to protect a person from some foreign invader and/or infectious agent, then fix it. Sounds so simple, doesn't it? The problem is, however, that so often the cause of inner bodily havoc is not known or understood.

There are so many different names for 80-100 autoimmune diseases, some very hard to pronounce. As autoimmunity is better understood as an etiology of disease, a person could simply say, "I have an autoimmune problem or illness," or "I suffer from disorderly autoimmunity." **Where** the cancer activity is denotes a specific site for cancer. **Where** the allergic or autoimmune reaction occurs, that may describe the location better, **but the cause of an autoimmune disease is still autoimmunity.**

"The common thread" in all of the autoimmune-related diseases, as Dr. Neil Rose, advisor for AARDA, would say is, of course, autoimmunity. This is what's important to understand. "The common etiology that brings together all of these diseases is autoimmunity." (37) Defining diseases by what causes the problem and developing action plans to counterattack the underlying reasons for a disease process, rather than simply treating the symptoms after the fact makes much more sense.

Yet to prevent something from occurring, the cause of the problem must first be the primary concern. We already know in the case of cancer, often the symptoms show up later, after the disease has time to continue for quite some time. Cancer treatment exists, but early detection is crucial and understanding and counteracting the cause of illness is imperative, not merely trying to fight the symptoms and allowing the essential trigger(s) of disease to continue.

Although, for some diseases, unfortunately, after a certain amount of damage is done, and for some conditions, management of inevitable symptoms, rather that prevention or a cure, is sometimes the only option. Quality of life is often obtained with health education and proper management of a disease. However, it still always helps to understand what causes a particular disease and symptoms, even if irreversible. And it's that understanding of the etiology of a disease which still offers the best chance for researchers to make progress toward preventive measures and cures. I once read in a pamphlet from National Jewish Hospital that "the key to conquering allergies and asthma, is understanding the diseases." I'm sure that's so true for all afflictions.

The fact that anti-inflammatory and immune-suppressive medications work to counteract or suppress the symptoms of autoimmunity and/or prevent damage means that if someone knows that autoimmunity is causing the problems, help is on the way. PERMANENT damage can be prevented! LIVES CAN BE SAVED! There is great potential for preventive medicine and preservation of quality of life, even life, with relation to autoimmune-related diseases. It's time to COUNTERATTACK, even prevent, the devastating effects of autoimmunity. With increased awareness, positive solutions, any necessary helpful lifestyle changes, and effective healthcare, tremendous progress and support will follow.

For those of us who fight the immunological wars within, we have already resolved to counterattack. We may be wounded and at times we are sick. But as Montel Williams professes, "WE ARE NOT WEAK!" We will not give up. We need soldier companions. Let us all work together against the terrorist attacks caused by inner immune-mediated wars responsible for so many hypersensitive and/or autoimmune-related casualties, as well as immune system deficiency-caused losses.

If auto (self) attack exists, then we can be certain that auto (self) counterattack is possible too. COUNTER-ATTACK! Let's make it a reality. Wars are tough, but we can win, now that we understand the enemy. Remember too, even with casualties of the past, present, or future—we always win, if we do not forget those who fought so bravely before us, and we never surrender our hopeful spirit.

Please note that in the entire book, I do address the issue about the controversies of vaccines. However, to open that "can of controversy' here would get me off track, so back to the epilogue for this book.

Finally, that monstrous disabling affliction—PAIN. It comes with the territory of autoimmune diseases and many neurological disorders. Because of chronic pain that zaps the life and functional abilities right out of a suffering person, those afflicted lose precious things. Oh they fight long and hard, but, like I said, PAIN is a monster, a thief. It steals and kills things that are precious to people such as: jobs, hobbies, functional and recreational abilities, families, lives, you name it—PAIN destroys it.

So, all I can do as someone who understands what it's like to endure pain is to offer: hope and support, encourage you to survive it, and thrive whenever possible, sometimes even overcome it. Also, I want to let pain sufferers know: "You are not alone," that's for sure. Take a ride with me down Pain Parkview Road. Maybe you'll feel a little better.

PAIN PARKVIEW ROAD

DEAR FELLOW CHRONIC PAIN SURVIVORS:

The late Emily Dickinson, gifted poet, wrote a poem about pain, something about how a person cannot remember when it started or if there was ever a pain-free time. Let's see if I can write a poem too. Guess it would go like this:

> PAIN, a debilitating monster,
> an It, that claims all joy within.
> From without, there may be no signs.
> But from within, hearts and minds
> are crushed by a toll so heavily
> that spirits may simply digress to dust,
> to the nothingness that only aches and rusts.
> To save ourselves, we must slay the monster,
> or at least be smarter than It.

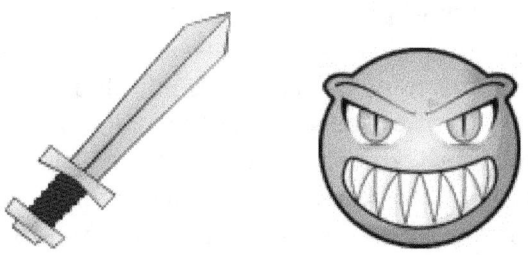

While driving down the road one day, a radio show host started talking to an author who had written a book about hpochondriasis or hypochondria, as we usually refer to the condition. It dawned on me, then and there, that fibromyalgia or the condition or syndrome which characterizes debilitating types of pain that cannot be detected with x-rays or other diagnostic tests is the perfect example of a modern day health crisis that many people deal with, try to endure, sometimes overcome, yet face being labeled a hypochondriac because there does not seem to be any proven reasons for pain.

Even with systemic lupus, there may have been many signs, symptoms, but the cause for some of the unnecessary deaths is because those afflicted may still "look" healthy. Yet, vital organs can be attacked, the pain worsens, bodily systems fail, and before a team of doctors even realizes the severity of the situation, it's too late, complications occur, and the patient sometimes dies. (My very first sad realization of this hit me when I read about the death of the actress Kellie Martin's 19 year old sister, Heather, due to lupus.)

Again, I appreciate the tremendous adaptive capabilities that human beings possess and certainly lifestyle choices are critical. But this notion that we can simply overcome anything and everything, that all disease is our fault, that pain is all about emotional problems, or that women just like to complain, etc., it's all got to stop. So often this type of thinking seems to pick up on adults and ignores the fact that millions of kids suffer diseases too and fight courageous battles to be as healthy as possible.

If you ever want to see some of these brave warriors for wellness, just surf the web for kids enduring juvenile rheumatoid arthritis and/or RA afflicted adults! I'm sorry, but just the right cup of "magic" tea isn't going to do it for them or millions of other children or adults fighting for their lives simply to enjoy a part of their day—pain-free.

What women, men, and children who deal with chronic pain need is this: first, a diagnosis which could simply be labeled as chronic and/or intermittent pain, then this incredibly empathetic approach, understanding, and reaction as noted by The American Academy of Pain Medicine.

"Each physician bears the responsibility to evaluate and treat persistent pain as a serious medical condition.

Principal treatment physicians must approach each patient with respect and urgency and provide appropriate and timely referrals to a Pain Medicine Specialist when primary medical care has not been effective." (38)   The consensus statement further explains: "Like many illnesses that at one time were not well understood, pain and its many manifestations may be poorly treated and seriously underestimated.   Inappropriately treated pain seriously compromises a patient's quality of life, causing emotional suffering and often leads to mood disorders, including depression and in rare cases, suicide." (39)

I don't know how people live with pain. (I don't know how I lived/live with it.) The best I can do though is try to offer hope, suggest a supportive family doctor, a pain specialist, and perhaps this: even if you've suffered for years, perhaps with understanding and effective rehabilitation, your health and life can improve. For those who have lost so much, no, you may not be able to return to the life you had; but there are always new beginnings, especially if the level of pain can be lowered to a more tolerable degree of hurt.

To the doctors and pain specialists who are there for us, I'll say this. Thanks for being there. So often the search is on for years and we never find you. Just one more important request. When we finally do find you, do us a favor. Before we do anything else and proceed to work hard again, (this time with some help), on improving our health, can we just sit down and spend one hour to talk, express our feelings, share our history, and have you listen and acknowledge how devastating it has been to try and survive? Like any war or concentration camp survivor, our wounds may not be visible, but they exist. If still suffering in severe pain, we are not really free yet.

My heart goes out to anyone afflicted with this disabling condition. Nobody wants this disabling affliction. Believe me, I'm sure I speak for all of us when I say, "We'd rather be pain-free and able to participate in life like anyone else." So many of the stories I've read regarding chronic pain survivors, they all worked before, they had co-workers, provided skills, one was a police officer, another a construction worker, many were nurses or wounded veterans. They all WANTED to continue working. They even tried and suffered for years to work part-time. After a while though, the wear and tear, the pain at one point, overwhelmed these victims, and a productive working life faded into a memory.

I detected hope for another chance over and over again. But as I said, the first hour of medical help in these cases should focus on one thing, an hour (well at least a half hour), of T.L.C. Like autoimmunity and hypersensitivity, the symptoms baffle, disrupt, cause havoc, maim, and kill. When pain happens, it's another affliction that must be counterattacked, as soon as possible, and with well-wishes that it's never too late.

Good luck with that most important balance beam, mind and immunity, immunity and the mind. No matter what afflictions, conflicts or crisis situations you encounter, counterattack! Kill the monsters of pain and adversity. Persevere and heal.*

Wellness hugs and God bless,

Gail Galvan

*Galvan, Gail M., L.P.N., B.A. Health and Wellness Education. *Autoimmunity Counterattack: A Sequel/The Healthy Road Back*. Montgomery, Alabama: www.e-booktime.com. (Letter is partial contents from pgs. 222-226 in my non-profit book.)

SUPPORTIVE SIDEWALKS

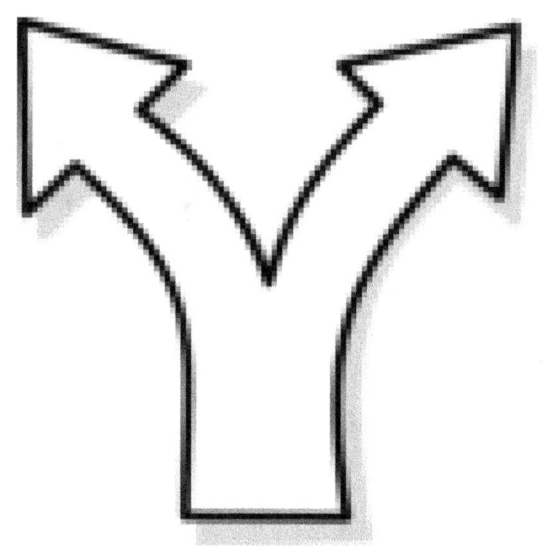

1. The Road Back Foundation (www.roadback.org)
2. www.RA-Infection-Connection.com
3. Dr. Gabe Mirkin (www.drmirkin.com)
4. www.rawarrior.com
5. The Arthritis Foundation (www.arthritis.org)
6. The Lupus Foundation of America (www.lupus.org)
7. The American Autoimmune-Related Disease Association (www.aarda.org)
8. The National Institute of Allergies and Infectious Diseases (www.niaid.nih.gov)
9. The Asthma and Allergy Foundation of America (www.aafa.org)
10. The American Academy of Pain Medicine (www.painmed.org)
11. The National Fibromyalgia Association (www.fmaware.org)
12. The John Hopkins Arthritis Center and Mayo Clinic
13. The Arthritis Center of Riverside, California (www.thearthritiscenter.com)
14. The National Multiple Sclerosis Society (www.nmss.org)
15. The National Institute of Arthritis and Musculoskeletal and Skin Diseases (www.niams.nih.gov)
16. The Arthritis Trust of America Foundation (www.arthritistrust.org)
17. The Alzheimer's Foundation of America since some research indicates possible inflammatory/autoimmunity causes (www.alzfd.org)
18. The American Lung Association (www.lung.org/lung-disease/asthma)
19. www.quackwatch.org Note: Opinions vary with this site. Many find it helpful to distinguish facts from fallacies/quackery in a complex world related to health, disease, and medicine. Others express concerns that the site sides with more conservative and/or orthodox treatments rather than acknowledging some research studies or the testimonials of many who claim that alternative choices have worked well. (Or inquire on a subject, check scam.)

Sadly, as Dr. Katherine Poehlmann suggests, the roads to wellness: prevention of and recovery from autoimmune and hypersensitivity afflictions are not smoothly paved or clearly lit. Though there may be more helpful pathways under construction than ever before, various avenues may have to be explored before the quickest, most beneficial direct routes to wellness and/or optimal health can be found. Keep following the sun—and in the darkness—keep your intuitive internal bright light turned on. Best of luck finding the healthy road back!

DOCTOR KATHERINE M. POEHLMANN

Dr. Katherine Poehlmann is the author of the recently published book: *Rheumatoid Arthritis: The Infection Connection {Targeting and Treating the Cause of Chronic Illness}*. This book describes the causes and antibiotic treatment of microbe-caused rheumatic diseases. In writing this book she has spent three years studying and correlating data on infectious organisms and chronic diseases. Her ongoing research includes examination of the link between Chlamydia and atherosclerosis. The slow-growing plaques clog arteries, resulting in unnecessarily high death rates from heart attacks and strokes among the elderly.

She is a professional researcher and a systems engineer with a magna cum laude degree in mathematics from Immaculate Heart College and an MBA from the University of Redlands with emphasis on technology management. She has authored more than a dozen scientific reports on space technology, defense policy analysis, and aircraft logistics.

Using her research skills, honed at the RAND Corporation as a senior analyst from 1984-1994, Katherine earned a Ph.D. in Health Science in 1997 after two years of intensive study. The goal was to find the cause of her own debilitating case of rheumatoid arthritis (RA) that developed in both of her ankles soon after a fall down stairs in 1993. She was told that RA was incurable, and that she would "just have to live with it." She saw that the usual course of treatment involved using powerful prescription drugs with harmful side effects. These medications only masked painful RA symptoms but did not target the root cause of her RA condition. She was determined to find a cure, if one existed.

DR. KATHERINE M. POEHLMANN (con't)

A turning point in her life was learning of the groundbreaking work by Dr. Thomas McPherson Brown in the 1940s that identified bacterial infection as an important factor in rheumatic disease. Her doctoral dissertation was the foundation for this book, significantly updated to include cutting edge advances in microbial infection research and more comprehensive coverage of chronic illnesses besides RA. Her self-help book is written for the lay person with a high school education, although Appendix II is written by a medical doctor *for* doctors so that they can clearly understand Dr. Brown's low dose, long term antibiotic protocol and its application for their patients.

Dr. Poehlmann progressed from being "25% disabled," as determined by four board-certified physicians and rheumatologists, to being completely ambulatory and pain-free within eight months, using the techniques described in this book. She also became a certified hypnotherapist in order to learn self-hypnosis techniques for stress control and pain management and teach them to others.

She was honored by the Torrance Cultural Arts Commission in April 2004 with the Excellence in Literary Arts Award.

Since recovery from RA, she has visited archeological sites in: Tibet, Chile, Easter Island, Malta, Ireland, Australia, and New Zealand and has hiked over sections of the Great Wall and Silk Route sites in China. Dr. Poehlmann lives in Torrance, CA and lectures widely on health topics. She waives speaker fees for community organizations, (i.e. Kiwanis), support groups, and library-sponsored events. All book profits, after expenses, are

DR. KATHERINE M. POEHLMANN (con't)

donated to infection research. Right brain (creative) talents include stand-up comedy and jewelry design. (On October 2, 2005, she performed at the Hollywood Improv.) For more information visit: www.AdornAgain.com and www.ra-infection-connection.com. (40)

Author's Note: I'd like to thank Dr. Poehlmann, again, for writing a foreword to my book and for her amazing dedication to helping others who must counterattack autoimmune afflictions.

DR. JATINDER K. KANSAL

Born: March 5, 1953 in the town of San Grur in Punjab, India

1975:   (Age 22) Graduated at age 22 from Government Medical College in Patiala, India. Earned an MB* and a B. S. (Bachelor of Medicine and Bachelor of Surgery)

College: Government Medical College in Patiala, India

1978:   (Age 25) Moved to the USA—Chicago, Illinois

1978-1981   Residency for 3 years of Post Graduate Training in Internal Medicine at Mercy Hospital, Chicago, Illinois

1981   Became Board Certified in Internal Medicine

1981-1983   Two year Fellowship under guidance of Doctor Samter at The Max Samter Institute of Allergy and Clinical Immunology, Grant Hospital, Chicago, Illinois

1983   Board Certified in Allergy and Immunology

1983   (Age 30) Obtained medical license in the state of Indiana and started own medical practice in Merrillville and Valparaiso, Indiana

2013   (Age 60) Dr. Kansal currently lives in Valparaiso, Indiana with his family and has offices in Valparaiso and Merrillville, Indiana

DOCTOR J. K. KANSAL (con't)

Dr. Kansal is married to Sadhna Kansal (35 yrs) and they have three children. Jay (a dentist), Seema (a Doctor in Internal Medicine), and Jagan, (a final year medical student).

"To the question, "What do you like to do in your spare time Dr. Kansal?"

He replied, "I love to walk, take nature walks, enjoy family, friends, and neighbors. I like reading, swimming, etc." (41)

*__Bachelor of Medicine, Bachelor of Surgery__, or in Latin:*__Medicinae Baccalaureus, Baccalaureus Chirurgiae__* (abbreviated in various ways, viz. *MBBS* or *MBChB, MB BS, MB BChir, BM BCh, MB BCh, MB ChB, BM BS, BM, BMed* etc.), are the two first professional undergraduate degrees awarded upon graduation from medical school in medicine and surgery by universities in various countries that follow the tradition of the United Kingdom. The naming suggests that they are two separate degrees; however, in practice, they are usually treated as one and awarded together. In countries that follow the tradition of the United States, the degree is awarded as M.D., which is a professional doctorate degree.[1] (42)

DOCTOR MAX SAMTER

Doctor Max Samter, in my opinion, should be considered the Louis Pasteur in relation to the medical field of allergy-related and immunological diseases. I found it odd that I had not run across his name before. Perhaps I did, but just forgot. Dr. Kansal had the pleasure of working under Dr. Samter's guidance for two years at The Max Samter Institute of Allergy and Clinical Immunology. When Dr. Kansal educated me about Dr. Samter's legacy, I really felt as if he belonged right here in this book, too. So here is a little history about him. Also, if you would like to read more about his fascinating life, how he liked motorcycles, and would sit and visit with patients for hours, check out a remarkable obituary about his important work and life at: https://jama.jamanetwork.com/article.aspx?articleid=19042 (44) Find the homepage at:http://jama.jamanetwork.com/journal.aspx.

Born: 1908 in Berlin, Germany.

1975-1983   Director of The Institute of Allergy and
                 Clinical Immunology at Grant Hospital
                 The Max Samter Institute of Allergy and
                 Clinical Immunology in Chicago, Illinois
                 was named in his honor.

Notable work: Samter's textbook, *Immunologic Diseases*,
                 was a forerunner and the 5th edition of his
                 book was published in 1995.

                 He is considered the most prolific medical
                 scientist in the area of Samter's Triad.

Died: 1999 in Evanston, Illinois (43)

SOURCES

NOTE: All glossary term information, with the exception of (mistaken identity,) was obtained by: http://en.wikipedia.org/wiki/Main_Page, the free online encyclopedia, Wikipedia. Information regarding (mistaken identify) was obtained by Dr. J. K. Kansal on (9-6-13). Thanks to both Dr. Kansal and Wikipedia for the resourceful information. For more in depth sources on any of numbered references, go to the Wikipedia page, enter the word/term, and you can research any sources further. For kids, another great resource to use in order to find more simplified definitions is: www.kids.net.au.

1. Galvan, Gail, *Autoimmunity Counterattack: A Sequel/The Healthy Road Back.* E-Booktime, LLC, Montgomery, Alabama, 2005, pgs. i-iii

2. Glasser, Ronald J., M.D., *The Body is the Hero.* New York: Bantam Books, 1979, p. 96.

3. Galvan, Gail, *Autoimmunity Counterattack: A Sequel/The Healthy Road Back.* E-Booktime, LLC, Montgomery, Alabama, 2005, p. 135.

4. http://aafa.org/display.cfm?id=9&sub=30

5. http://aafa.org/display.cfm?id=8&sub=42

6. http://www.niaid.nih.gov/news/newsreleases/2012/Pages/WorldAsthmaDay2012.aspx

7. American Autoimmune Disease Related Associations. (AARDA) "Autoimmunity, A Major Women's Health Issue." Pamphlet.

SOURCES (con't)

8. Ibid.
9. Ibid.
10. Ibid.
11. Ibid.
12. Ibid.
13. Ibid.
14. Ibid.
15. Ibid.

16. Lupus Foundation of America, Northwest Indiana Chapter, Portage, Indiana. *Orientation to Lupus*, second edition, April 2000, p.2.

17. Ibid.
18. Ibid.
19. Ibid.
20. Ibid.
21. Ibid.
22. http://activebiotech.com/research-areas

23. Rheumatoid Arthritis Pamphlet, www.arthritis.org

24. Ibid.
25. Ibid.
26. Ibid.
27. Ibid.
28. Ibid.
29. Ibid.

30. Cantwell Jr., Alan, Dr., "Tetracycline for RA: Is it Safe?"pgs.1-2 http://www.roadback.org/index.cfm? fuseaction=ecuation.display&display_id=116

SOURCES (con't)

31. Ibid.
32. Ibid.

33. AARDA, "Autoimmunity, A Major Women's Health Issue," pamphlet.

34. Ibid.

35. Meadows, Michelle. "Understanding Vaccine Safety: Immunization Remains Our Best Defense Against Deadly Disease," http:/www.fda.gov/fdac/features/2001/401_vacc.

36. AARDA. "What Do These Diseases Have in Common? Autoimmunity." Pamphlet.

37. Rose, Noel R., M.D., Ph.D., "Autoimmunity-The Common Thread," http:www.aarda.org/commonthread, AARDA InFocus Article, p. 2.

38. http://www.painmed.org/ Workarea/DownloadAsset.aspx?id=3207American Academy of Pain.
   .

39. Ibid.

40. http://www.ra-infection-connection.com (About the Author)

41. Dr. J.K. Kansal (9-13-13).

42. http://en.wikipedia.org/wiki/Bachelor_of_Medicine

SOURCES (con't)

43. http://www.en.wikipedia.org/wiki/Max_Samter

44. Asthma and Allergy Foundation of America. "Allergist of the Year." *Advance* (Greater Chicago Chapter Newsletter) Autumn 1982: Vol. 11, No. 1.

Author's Websites:

Google: gail galvan books

https://gailgalvanbooks.wordpress.com/

https://gailgalvanbooks.wordpress.com/gail-galvan-podcast/

www.newjackrabbitcity.podomatic.com

new jack rabbit city the trailer

Contact author at:
ggpodbooks@hotmail.com
savesoulusa@gmail.com

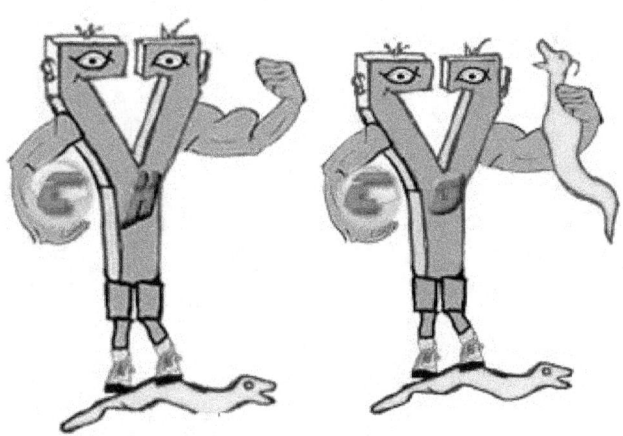

TO VIEW A VIDEO WHICH
SHOWS THE AUTHOR DEMONSTRATING
CAPABILITIES WITH MEDICATIONS AND
THE DEVASTATING EFFECTS
(INCAPABILITIES) WITHOUT MEDS FOR
HER AUTOIMMUNE DISEASE

VISIT YOUTUBE AT:
rheumatoid arthritis video diary.

"So often we look healthy when we see doctors,
but take away the meds, and the disabling flare-ups
SHOW, don't tell, a painfully different picture!
Good luck fellow survivors!" GG